Dick Gregory's
Natural Diet
for Folks Who Eat

Dick Gregory's Natural Diet for Folks Who Eat

Cookin' with Mother Nature

Dick Gregory

Edited by James R. McGraw with Alvenia M. Fulton

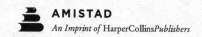
AMISTAD
An Imprint of HarperCollins*Publishers*

Excerpts on pages 66–68 and 81–86 are adapted from *Diet and Salad Suggestions* (1971 edition), by N. W. Walker (Phoenix, Arizona: Norwalk Press), and are used here with the kind permission of the author.

First Perennial Library edition published in 1974
First Amistad paperback published in 2021

Designed by Terry McGrath

Library of Congress Cataloging-in-Publication Data has been applied for.

ISBN 978-0-06-298141-7

24 25 26 27 28 LBC 8 7 6 5 4

TO MOTHER NATURE
and her faithful children—
nutritionists, naturopaths, life
extensionists, chiropractors, and
all others loving the natural way
of life—who have persevered through years
of ridicule, rejection and scorn and
found their reward in "cookin' with
Mother Nature"

Contents

Dick Gregory's Natural Diet for Folks Who Eat

Editor's Note

Readers who are considering adopting the raw-juice therapy, fasting or other dietary regimens suggested in this book should be advised that what works for some will not work for others. Anyone considering a diet should first consult his or her physician, particularly anyone with a special medical problem.

1

Warning: The Author Has Determined That Not Reading the Following Pages Is Dangerous to Your Health

This is a book for folks who are willing to take time to stop and think. I've often said that one of the biggest problems in America today is that we Americans just don't think, not just about food—about anything.

The trouble with us Americans is that we've never thought. Remember that old cleanser commercial? "Keep the rust out of the entire house!" So folks would clean up all the rusty spots. But if they ever thought to pick up that can of cleanser after it had been sitting for a while, sure enough they'd have found that little brown rusty ring!

Let's take another example. We spend millions of dollars in the United States every year for civil defense buildings. But do you realize most of them are *closed on weekends*? It's as if we think our enemies are planning to fight a five-day war! Even Israel took six days.

Life insurance is another good example. Probably no other group of people on the face of this earth spends more money on life insurance than we do in the United States. Did you ever stop and think that you have to be slightly stupid to buy life insurance? But just analyze this. You're betting the insurance company people that you're going to die. And they're betting you that you are going to live. And you're hoping they win. And *they* charge *you*.

Sometimes the strangest things cause you to stop and think. I remember when I first started thinking about whether or not it was right to eat meat. It was on Thanksgiving Day a number of years ago. I had been drinking while I waited for the turkey to get done. It takes a turkey a long time. By the time I was standing at the head of the table with my carving knife, I suddenly had the strangest thoughts. I got to thinking that there might be some beings on another planet somewhere who are as intelligent compared with us as we are compared with turkeys.

Now that's a disturbing thought! I could just see myself in some strange planetary oven, being basted and roasted. It would be one thing to roast white folks brown; they'd be trying to figure out a way to "undone" us black folks. I even thought about myself lying on a platter all filled with stuffing!

Then I had visions of these beings from another planet going to the butcher shop with their meat list. I wonder what they'd call their butcher shops? They'd probably call them "folks shops." I could hear them placing an order: "Give me a half dozen Oriental knees, two Caucasian feet and twelve fresh Black lips." And the folks-shopkeeper comes back smiling and says, "These Black lips are so fresh they're still talkin'." After that little fantasy, I couldn't eat my Thanksgiving dinner. But it started me thinking.

There would be a whole lot of changes in America if we Americans decided one day to start thinking. And one of the biggest and most important changes would be in the "traditional" American diet. The old saying is very true: "You are what you eat." It would be more accurate, perhaps, to say: "You are what you assimilate." That is, your body literally is what you assimilate from the "foods"—or more frequently "things"—you eat to rebuild cells and what you eliminate as waste products of the cell-building activity as you revitalize yourself each day.

If you just stop and look around you, you can see—and many of you can *feel*—the sorry results of the eating habits of the majority of folks in America today. Folks getting old twenty, thirty, forty or even fifty years before their time. Swollen ankles, varicose veins, pot bellies, bald heads, arthritis, rheumatism, ulcers, sinus trouble, eye trouble, mental illness, gallstones, prostate gland trouble, hemorrhoids, heart trouble, liver trouble, kidney trouble, overweight, underweight, anemia, bad feet, headaches, short breath, can't sleep or can't wake up, no energy, "tired" blood, sitting in front of the television set all evening and falling asleep watching it—the list is endless and very, very familiar.

Dr. Laura Newman, in her 1970 book *Make Your Juicer Your Drugstore,* reports: "During the last 50 years in the U.S.A., the increase of Epilepsy has been 450%; Diabetes, 1800%; Bright's Disease, 650%; Anemia, 300%; Insanity, 400%; Heart Trouble, 300%; Cancer, 308%; and, while we have the distinction of raising the world's best hogs, we have 75% of the world's Sinus Trouble."

The sad truth is that all of these afflictions, and their unbelievable increase, are the result of Americans' habit of putting "garbage" in their stomach instead of in the disposal. Most folks throw leftover garbage in the incinerator, disposal or garbage can—but only after they have tossed down or gulped—seldom chewed!—the greatest percentage of garbage into their own bodies.

It is very hard to unlearn the falsehoods we have accepted

as truth all our lives. So much of what we are taught—both in school and at our mother's knee—is nothing more than accepted, handed-down opinion that simply will not hold up under cold, hard analysis or weather the test of new experience. The great scientist Albert Einstein described most of what we learn as "a collection of prejudices which are fed to us with a porridge spoon before our eighteenth year." In schools at all grade levels, teachers present the current theories and notions of the time as though they were established facts. But the passage of time, combined with new experience and research, makes yesterday's "facts" today's myths, superstitions and falsehoods.

Einstein's description is uniquely appropriate when it comes to the matter of personal diet. We are *literally* spoon fed wrong food and wrong notions about what we ought to eat! It begins when we are babies and food is inserted in our mouths; we are offered no choice. For many of us the process never changes! The only alternative babies have is to spit it out—which of course they often do. Mothers see that reaction as something babies go through until they learn how to eat rather than as the natural response of innocence to a violation of Mother Nature's rules!

Teachers in the great centers of education in the ancient world (e.g., Pythagoras at Crotona) were very hip. They understood that it was impossible for folks to *learn* anything until they had *experienced its truth for themselves.* So the ancient teachers set up a curriculum where their pupils *practiced* the arts of numerology and dynamic geometry, for example, to *experience* the faculty of intuition. From that experience a pupil could go on to apprehend the essential laws of cosmic motion.

This book is based upon that ancient understanding of how we learn. The book grew out of my own personal experience. Its pages reflect what I have learned—what I have experienced as Truth and what I hope you will try for yourself—in my new life of "cookin' with Mother Nature."

Unless you are already very heavy into the natural-food-and-way-of-life movement, most of what you read in *Natural Diet for Folks Who Eat* will go against everything you've ever believed about food, eating, health and disease. I can only say to you, "Don't feel too bad. I started out on an equal footing with the worst-eatin' reader of these pages!"

But I was fortunate. I met a teacher in the "ancient tradition," Dr. Alvenia M. Fulton. I'll speak more of her later, but in this chapter I'll just testify! When I met her, Dr. Fulton was confident that she possessed the truth about food, nutrition and proper diet. But she also knew I would have to experience that Truth for myself. I resisted every step of the way. Out of ignorance, I argued, rationalized and repeated all the wrong notions about food I had been taught.

Why? Because I just couldn't believe my momma would have fed me meat if it was wrong, or given me cow's milk if it was wrong. And here was a stranger, a woman I had just met, telling me that my own momma had fed me wrong! My momma never had the benefit of learning the Truth about proper diet, and as a result she suffered many of the physical results of improper eating habits. We were very poor and my momma's main concern was that we kids got "somethin' to eat."

Every time I would come up with one of my stupid arguments, trying to refute what Dr. Fulton was telling me about some new way to change my diet, she would smile and say, "Just try it for me. Try it for a while and see what happens." I tried it, and invariably I liked it! I liked the fresh, pure tastes of natural foods; but even more important, I liked the glowing feeling of health, vigor and energy which followed my change in diet.

So many times I hear people resist changing their diet because they don't want to *give up something they like.* That's the first great myth to be dispelled. Learning to eat as Mother Nature intended her children to eat does not mean giving up something. It means just the opposite! It means *gaining* something of great value— a value far greater than the old rationalization "I've grown accustomed to its taste." It means gaining health, youthful energy and appearance, increased mental capacity, and a joy in living you never dreamed was possible. To say nothing of the clean, fresh, natural taste of the food you will be enjoying!

The more I tried out Dr. Fulton's recommendations, the more I began to realize the sad neglect of my formal education. I had gone the whole school route—grade school, high school and college—and never once did I take a course in "Nature." I was never taught that the most important thing in life was learning to live in harmony with Nature. My formal education was so designed to teach me *how to make a living,* it never got around to teaching me *how to live*! I was taught about so-called civilization's attempt to *control* Nature and about the ongoing war *against* Nature (although those terms were never used). I learned about the industrial revolution, the invention of the automobile, the steam engine and the airplane, the world wars, the atomic bomb and the hydrogen bomb, and other "accomplishments" of twentieth-century civilization. I was taught about great thinkers, great political and military leaders, great philosophies and ideologies, but none of them told me about Nature.

But Mother Nature herself is a great teacher. She provides *experience.* And our experience reminds us over and over again, "It's not nice to fool Mother Nature!"

Fool around with Mother Nature's clouds, "seeding" them and conducting other experiments, and eventually you will have a "natural disaster" on your hands—a flood or hurricane. Absorb enough alcohol in your bloodstream and sooner or later Mother Nature's liver will go on strike and your body declare a work stoppage. Expel enough smoke, exhaust and fumes into the air and eventually Mother Nature's respiratory system will show you what you can do with all that "progress." Eat bad enough, long enough, and Mother Nature will send you little notes of reprimand—tooth decay, high blood pressure, heart trouble, kidney trouble or any of the other ways she uses to remind us "It's not nice." Try to fool Mother Nature and she will make a fool out of you!

Rather than trying to exercise "control," a truly civilized humanity should try to learn enough *self-control* to live in happy harmony with Mother Nature.

I want to share with you my new experiences with Mother Nature. Hopefully you'll learn something *and* have a few smiles. But most important is the experience you will gain in living a more natural way of life—the joyful experience of "cookin' with Mother Nature."

2

From Omnivore to Fruitarian in Seven Short Years

The Continuum of Consumption

Diet, or systems of eating, may be viewed as a continuum, a straight line running between two extremes—eating *everything* and eating *nothing*. All along the line are major stopping-off points, stages of diet which set limitations on what may properly be consumed. I have moved from one extreme to the other on the "Continuum of Consumption." Seven years ago I began my present dietary journey as a confirmed omnivore. And now I am a fruitarian.

Omnivorism, at one extreme of the Continuum of Consumption, involves eating everything. Most people begin at this point and stay there all their lives. It's the "official" diet of so-called civilized humanity.

Omnivores eat cooked food and they eat raw food, though they seem to prefer their poison heated. They eat fruits, vegetables, grains, cereals (usually in the form of devitalized breakfast foods), breads (mostly white), cakes, pies, beef, pork, poultry, lamb, fish, beans, nuts, cheese, eggs, pizza and chitterlings! They broil their steaks on the backyard barbecue, or they eat their meat raw and appropriately name the barbaric dish tartar steak.

Of course, omnivores may impose certain restrictions on their diet. Some call a halt to *escargots* when they find they are eating snails. Others pass by such delicacies as chocolate-covered ants, grasshoppers or octopus. But for most omnivores, *everything* is fair game for consumption, and they are limited only by personal preference.

When I was an omnivore, a favorite nightclub routine illustrated one limitation I imposed upon my diet. I would tell of walking into a restaurant down South. I sat down and picked up the menu. Pretty soon the waitress came over to me and said, "We don't serve colored people here!" I looked up innocently and said, "That's all right, ma'am, I don't eat 'em!" But outside of *that* matter of personal taste, anything got past me.

Vegetarianism, more properly called lacto-vegetarianism, consists of eating only plant substances (fruits, vegetables, grains, cereals, nuts, etc.), along with milk, milk products, eggs and honey.

Unlike omnivores, vegetarians will not eat flesh. They follow a nonflesh diet for humanitarian or health reasons, or a combination of both.

It begins to look like President Nixon is adding another reason to the list of points in favor of vegetarianism—the *price* of food, especially of meat. My brother, who's still a meat-eater, went into the supermarket the other day and he had to buy his T-bone steak on the layaway plan. I understand food prices are so high that on the last moon shot the astronauts had to give up their Tang for Kool-Aid!

Because of food prices, I've noticed a different reaction from people over the past few months. In fact, people used to think I was crazy following the kind of diet I do and fasting so much, but now folks don't ask me *why* I fast. They ask how *they* can do it. If the price of food gets any higher, Nixon will have more people on fasts than Gandhi!

Veganism is the exclusion of all animal substances from the diet. Vegans reject milk, cheese, eggs and all foods coming from animals. That, of course, would include Jell-O and other gelatins, since they come from animal hoofs. Strict vegans would need to be careful about taking vitamin pills to make sure they are not swallowing a gelatin capsule.

Apart from considerations of what a person should or should not eat for health reasons, veganism is based upon the moral conviction that human beings must get things right between themselves and the animal kingdom. Vegans deplore the evil treatment animals receive at the hands of humans, including such activities as hunting, fishing, fur trading, and such places of animal exploitation as slaughterhouses, henhouses, breeding pens, scientific experimental laboratories and circuses.

Vegan writers, like Alfred Hy. Haffenden, often refer to the Day of Judgment, when the Creator will hold humankind accountable for its relationship to the animal kingdom. Every time I pass a Colonel Sanders Kentucky Fried Chicken stand, I have the same thought. Wouldn't it be wild if Colonel Sanders got to Heaven one day and found out God was a chicken? If that ever happens, I sure hope I'm standing there right behind the Colonel. I'd whisper in his ear, "Go on and tell Chicken Big he's 'finger-lickin' good.'"

Vitarianism excludes all animal substances *and* plant seeds from the diet. Vitarians go a step beyond vegans and rule out grains, legumes, nuts and all actual seeds. Those who are vitarians by religious conviction believe that plant seeds were not intended by God for human consumption. They also feel that eating seeds has stimulated the "seed principle" in human beings, making them slaves to sex and sensual living. Perhaps that explains why nuts are usually served in cocktail lounges and at parties!

Fruitarianism is the eating of fruit alone. Fruitarians—I am now one of them—believe that Mother Nature intended her children to be *frugivorous*, or fruit-eating. And whether the Holy Bible or the theory of evolution is your particular scripture, there is good reason to accept the fruitarian point of view.

In the Bible, chapter 1, verse 29 of the Book of Genesis says: "And God said, 'Behold, I have given you every plant yielding seed which is upon the face of all the earth, and every tree with seed in its fruit; you shall have them for food'" (RSV). The King James version translates the same verse somewhat differently: "And God said, Behold, I have given you every herb bearing seed, which is upon the face of all the earth, and every tree, in the which is the fruit of a tree yielding seed; to you it shall be for *meat*." (Italics mine.)

So the story of creation in the Bible says that fruit is the food human beings are divinely intended to eat and that "meat-eating" means a fruitarian diet rather than consuming the flesh of animals! And the physical makeup of human beings supports this understanding of divine creation. People have more in common with the frugivorous than the *carnivorous*, or flesh-eating, members of the animal kingdom.

First of all, flesh-eating animals have a very short intestinal tract. This is necessary because of the highly putrefactive character of the food they eat, namely flesh, or "meat" in the nonbiblical sense of the word. Human beings, on the other hand, have very *long* intestinal tracts, so it should seem obvious that Mother Nature never intended a meat diet for people. We just don't have the guts for it, so to speak. We shall see later the problems suffered by meat-eating humans when constipation prevents proper elimination and the waste products of a flesh diet remain where they don't belong.

Secondly, carnivorous animals are provided with special teeth to seize their prey and tear the flesh from them. Human beings, like apes and chimpanzees, lack such dental equipment. Apes, for example, could never manage eating the carcasses of large animals, nor could humans until they invented knives and forks! A look at the teeth of human beings shows they were intended to eat pulpy fruits, succulent stems and leaves rather than flesh.

Finally, the digestive juices of human beings indicate that Mother Nature did not intend her human children to be carnivorous. The digestion of flesh requires great amounts of hydrochloric acid, which is supplied in concentrated form in the bodies of carnivorous animals. If humans were intended to eat meat, they would have acids sufficient to digest bone as well as flesh.

So fruitarians are content to accept the word of scripture and physical evidence and consume only fruit, direct from plants and trees, in a natural state, fully "cooked" by Mother Nature's outdoor oven—sun, light, air and moisture. Only fruits and flowers are so directly exposed to Mother Nature's solar energies.

The final extreme of the continuum is *"breathatarianism,"* or "eating nothing." It is living entirely on a transcendental plane, breathing in pure air, absorbing the direct light and energies of the sun, bathing in pure water—in other words, living on what some writers call the "supersubstantial bread." I personally believe breathatarianism to be the highest mode of human living and an entirely possible way of life under ideal circumstances.

Charles Atlas Revisited

At the time of this writing, I weigh about 97 pounds—a near 200 percent reduction from my former weight—and of course, being a 97-pounder has its effect upon race relations, as it has upon many other experiences. I've lost so much weight that non-violence is no longer a tactic, it's a necessity!

My current weight reminds me of the old magazine ads for the Charles Atlas body-building course. In case your memory needs refreshing, the ad was a cartoon strip which began with a picture of a skinny "97-pound weakling" lying on a blanket on the beach with his girl friend. Along comes a muscular, bulging-biceped bully who kicks sand in the skinny one's face and challenges him to do something about it. The poor weakling is clobbered, and the girl walks off with the bully, somehow having been "turned on" by the unprovoked display of violence!

The dejected weakling returns to his bedroom—alone—and begins a crash body-building program under the mail order direction of Charles Atlas. In a very few weeks, the weakling builds up his physique, returns to the same beach, beats hell out of the same bully and gets back the same girl.

I guess you would have to say I am the antithesis of that ad. I became a 97-pounder by choice, having shed almost 200 pounds to get that way. And while a desire to be successfully violent inspired the weakling in the ad to build himself up, it was an *aversion* to violence and killing in all forms that initiated my slimming down. Now that I know more about proper diet, I think back on the Charles Atlas ad and realize the bully was probably a heavy meat-eater, egged on to "manly" pursuits by the poison in his system.

I was born and raised in the ghetto of Saint Louis and like most black families, mine was large and poor. Living in a large, poor family posed problems. For example, there were so many of us kids sleeping in the same bed, if I got up to go to the bathroom in the middle of the night, I had to leave a bookmark so I wouldn't lose my spot! We were so poor that one time we got garnisheed by the newspaper boy!

Even though we were poor, I remember once a year my daddy would save up some money, pack up all us kids, and take us out to dinner. Our family was so big, every year it would cost him $125—and that was at a ten-cent hamburger stand! Holidays posed special problems. We never had enough food. I remember one Thanksgiving when my momma came home with a turkey foot. All of us kids gathered around the pot while Momma boiled the foot, and we watched it shrink. Then we all sat at the table looking at the turkey foot and waiting to dive into it, and Momma insisted that we pray over it first! I told her, "Momma, I don't have anything against prayers or anything like that. But if anyone ought to be praying, it should be the turkey that got away from that foot."

About the only holiday we could enjoy was Halloween. Halloween was the one day in the year we could wear our regular clothes and people thought we were dressed for the occasion. Every Halloween, when I went to get my meal by trick or treat, folks would look at me and say, "Look at Richard wearing that old man's costume. And he's wearing shoes that look just like feet!"

As a kid, I was always *obsessed* with food, with good reason. The nutritional concern in our home was always *quantity* rather than *quality* of food. It's part of the insecurity of being poor. Now I have learned that the less food a person eats the better, as long as it is the right kind of food and it composes a balanced diet. But in a poor household, where there is always the possibility of no food at all, the tendency is to *overreact* when food is present.

At mealtime I was always encouraged to be an omnivore. Momma would say, "Eat everything on your plate!" Being hungry had nothing to do with it, just as hunger never told us *when* to eat. If it was "mealtime" and there was food in the house, we ate it.

Insecurity about food will never allow poor folks to turn down food. Not only is the worry ever present that one day there may be no food at all, but poor folks tend to believe the myth that the more food you eat, the better nourished and more healthy you will be. A fat person is well fed, or "healthy." It would not occur to most poor folks that a person who is fat is probably suffering from malnutrition!

As I look back at my childhood, I realize I was a "junkie." Most of my diet consisted of junk—candy, Pepsi-Cola with salted peanuts, Twinkies, cupcakes, doughnuts, cookies, popcorn at the movies, whatever I could get my hands on and my teeth into. In those early days of my youth, I didn't eat "soul food" as much as "stole food." I fed myself out of my own pocket—whatever I could steal or earn.

Actually, some of the food I got *inside* my home as a kid started out as "stole food" and became "soul food." My momma would bring home food she got by raiding the pantry of the white folks she worked for, and she'd cook it up.

Since canned foods were too expensive for poor folks, most of the vegetables I ate as a kid were fresh, but they were always cooked. The meat was usually fried. The only time we kids ate fresh fruit was when we were sick. I used to think of fresh fruit as medicine, the same as cod liver or castor oil, and would therefore reject it. Now I know that fresh fruit and vegetables—and their juices—are the best medicine in the world.

When I went to the restaurant or lunch counter to feed myself out of my own pocket, I never ordered a regular meal. I always had a bowl of chili and a hamburger, or a hot dog. At the Chinese restaurant it was always fried pork and rice.

I would say about 80 percent of everything I ate as a kid fell into the "junk" category. And I suffered because of it, but until I learned more about nutrition I never knew why. I had severe rheumatism, arthritis, stomach and sinus trouble as a kid. Sometimes the pain was so bad I would lie in bed at night and cry, all knotted up in a ball. It never dawned on me then that Mother Nature was talking to me!

My diet improved somewhat when I became interested in track in high school and I tried to lay off the "junk" diet. And when I got to college, on a track scholarship, my diet improved even more. I ate more regular, balanced meals than ever before, though even the "educated" college kitchen was ignorant of Mother Nature's teaching.

When I left college and settled down in Chicago to try and make it on my own, I reverted. The wolf was at my door once more. I concentrated on how to earn some rent money and survive—and by this time I had added alcohol and cigarettes to my omnivorous diet.

January 13, 1961, was the beginning of my Steak Career. People who have read the story of my life may remember that date as the night of my Big Break in show business. I was called into Chicago's Playboy Club that evening to fill in for the regular comedian, Prof. Irwin Corey. It turned out that the room had been booked by a convention of *frozen food* executives from the deep South, and when I arrived at the club the management suggested I consider not going on. But I decided to go on anyway, and after some very tense opening moments, I won over the crowd, got a standing ovation and scored a huge success. From that night on I could eat anything.

The "best" restaurants replaced candy stores, lunch counters and delicatessens. I was still feeding myself out of my own pocket, but that pocket was much fuller now, and I could eat all the meals I never had as a kid. I was wealthy enough to buy the richest meals in the most expensive eating places, and I was determined to satisfy every taste I ever had.

I was realizing an omnivore's dream. I would go into a restaurant and say, "Give me everything!" I never made a choice between items on a menu. I'd just order three, four, five or six dinners—whatever attracted my eye and excited my taste buds. Often my table at a restaurant looked like a combination ocean and barnyard, as the waiter delivered lobster, steak, chicken, pork chops and barbecued ribs in a single serving. Not that I would eat every bite. Few of the best omnivores could have pulled that off! But I stuffed myself and made sure I satisfied every taste.

I ate as much as and as often as I wanted. I would eat as many times a day as time permitted or inclination suggested. I ate regular meals and between-between-meal snacks. I continued to smoke three or four packs of cigarettes a day, and I washed it all down with a daily fifth of Scotch.

By the old standards of my ghetto youth, I should have been "healthy." I was "well fed," which meant I ate a lot. I got fatter and fatter. I wore suits with double-breasted vests which stylishly covered my expanding belly. But even the best of fashion was no comfort when I sat down; on an airplane I always unbuttoned the waist of my pants before fastening my seat belt. But I wasn't healthy, of course. Far from it. I still had my excruciatingly painful stomach trouble and my bad sinuses.

It is very strange how food and career have crisscrossed in my life. That convention of frozen food execs at the Playboy Club started me on the road to fame in show business. My new status led to my first involvement in the civil rights movement of the 1960s. And the philosophy of nonviolence which I learned from Dr. Martin Luther King, Jr., during my involvement in the civil rights movement was first responsible for my change in diet.

I became a vegetarian in 1965. I had been a participant in all of the "major" and most of the "minor" civil rights demonstrations of the early sixties, including the March on Washington and the Selma to Montgomery March. Under the leadership of Dr. King, I became totally committed to nonviolence, and I was convinced that nonviolence meant opposition to killing in any form. I felt the commandment "Thou shalt not kill" applied to human beings not only in their dealings with each other—war, lynching, assassination, murder and the like—but in their practice of killing animals for food or sport. Animals and humans suffer and die alike. Violence causes the same pain, the same spilling of blood, the same stench of death, the same arrogant, cruel and brutal taking of life.

One night, during a nightclub engagement in San Francisco, while sitting in a hotel room in the wee hours of the morning talking with my comedy writer Jim Sanders, I made the decision never to eat meat again. I had become firmly convinced that the killing of animals for food was both immoral and unnatural. Human beings are the most beautifully and brilliantly constructed machines in the universe. They are endowed by Nature with a wisdom and an intelligence surpassed by no other creature. As a human being and the beneficiary of Mother Nature's endowment of mind and body, I refused to accept that I had to stoop to the lowliness of *killing* something to get my dinner.

It was a moral decision. It had nothing to do with an understanding of proper diet. I had no desire to lose weight. And I still smoked my three or four packs of cigarettes a day and drank my fifth of Scotch.

If it is possible to be an "omnivorous vegetarian," I was it! I ate everything in the vegetable line, mostly cooked vegetables. I would go into a soul food restaurant and wipe out the yams, greens, black-eyed peas, macaroni and cheese, corn bread, squash, dressing—everything on the menu but the meat dishes.

For a short while I continued to eat Jell-O, until I realized it came from animal hoofs, and you usually have to kill animals to get them to give up their hoofs. So I stopped eating Jell-O, which was hard to do. When I was younger I used to have a Jell-O habit. When I couldn't get it, I'd lie in the gutter and shake!

I still followed, in *quantity* and *frequency*, the eating pattern of my Steak Career, and my weight jumped up more than a hundred pounds. I had weighed about 167 pounds when I became a vegetarian, and I reached a top weight of 288.

All of a sudden I was aware that another change had taken place in my body. My stomach trouble and my sinus trouble had disappeared! The only thing that was different about my way of life was that I no longer ate meat. So I was convinced that meat was responsible for my stomach and sinus ailments. If I had stopped smoking or stopped drinking when I became a vegetarian, I would have sworn the alcohol or tobacco was responsible for my physical problems.

My next major change in diet came in 1967. That spring I ran as the independent write-in candidate for mayor of Chicago. Mayor Richard Daley was my most formidable opponent, and when the votes were counted, Mayor Daley had received enough of an edge to win another term. When you say the votes are counted in Chicago, you really mean it. They are counted, and counted, and counted. In Chicago, you seldom hear of a candidate on Mayor Daley's machine ticket demanding a recount. The chances are the candidate's votes have *already* been recounted, several times, added up, and all the recounts reported as the total vote! Chicago's the only city in the country where, on election night, the national television networks show reruns! The 1972 elections were a blow to the Daley machine in Chicago. For example, Daniel Walker, an anti-machine candidate, won the election for governor. Governor Walker first came to national attention when he issued a commission report after the 1968 Democratic Convention in Chicago saying the Chicago police *rioted.* After the '72 elections, I wouldn't have been surprised to see Mayor Daley issue a report saying the Chicago voters did the same thing!

But I campaigned hard in 1967 and made a point. My candidacy for mayor of Chicago (and my later write-in candidacy for president of the United States in 1968) was intended to illustrate that in a democracy the voters should have not only the right to *elect* but also the right to *select.* Usually the voters have only the opportunity to choose between candidates someone else has already named to be on the ballot. A voter who wrote my name on the ballot was holding a nominating convention and casting a vote at the same time.

During my campaign for mayor, a lady stopped by my campaign headquarters while I was out on the streets and dropped off salads for my staff and myself. Since I was not there, she left her name—Dr. Alvenia Fulton—and her address.

When I returned I refused to eat the salad, since I didn't know Dr. Fulton and was suspicious of anybody I didn't know trying to feed me something while I was campaigning to overthrow the Daley machine! I was afraid someone might be trying to poison me.

A few months after the election, I told my wife, Lillian, we really should go by and see that lady who sent the salads to campaign headquarters. We did, and our conversations began.

As I said before, food and career have strangely crisscrossed in my life. It is the same with my "career" in social protest. When I first became involved in the civil rights movement, people used to ask me, "Have demonstrations hurt your career?" I always answered, "The proper question is, 'Has my career got in the way of demonstrations?'"

My *career* involves my work as a comedian, lecturer, author, recording artist, television and film personality. My *vocation* involves my participation in the struggle for human dignity—the human rights movement. The increased knowledge of proper diet has accompanied my deeper understanding of my vocation. My vocation, which began in the *civil* rights movement, has now been expanded to include the *human* rights and peace movements. Thus, my expanded vocation led to the next major change in my diet.

In talking with Dr. Fulton, I kept hearing of the beneficial aspects of fasting. Like most people, I was afraid to go on a long fast. All my life I had been told, "If you don't eat, you'll die." I had read about Gandhi's fasts, and I greatly admired the man, but his dedication and commitment was a lesson from history rather than a shared experience.

I wanted to do something dramatic and personal to protest the continued slaughter in Vietnam. Dr. Fulton had fasted many times, and she had prescribed fasts for her patients. I became more and more convinced I, too, should go on a long fast, at least thirty days. So I decided, in the latter days of 1967, to take only distilled water for nourishment, beginning Thanksgiving Day and continuing until New Year's Day, 1968. My fast was for moral reasons, as a social protest.

Dr. Fulton must have sensed my uneasiness with the decision. She told me, "If you're really serious about this fast, I'll go on it with you." She did. Not only did she fast right along with me, but she guided and counseled me every step of the way. She told me how to prepare for the fast by cleaning out my body. She put me on a diet of fruit juice seven days prior to Thanksgiving, and she told me to cleanse my colon with enemas and to continue the enemas after the fast began. Under the direction of Dr.

Fulton, what started out as a kind of "hunger strike" became a "scientific fast."

That first fast was the experience of my life! I started out weighing 280 pounds and on New Year's Day I was under a hundred pounds. I had become that "97-pound weakling," but felt stronger and healthier than ever before. I maintained my usual hectic schedule throughout the fast, traveling to fifty-seven cities in forty days. I gave sixty-three lectures.

On the weekends preceding Christmas I worked the Village Gate nightclub in New York City, doing three shows a night. It was at the Gate that one of the funniest incidents of my first fast occurred. Well into my performance, I had got up from the stool I usually use in my act and was pacing back and forth across the stage, microphone in hand. At one point I made a dramatic gesture, swinging my arm away from my body suddenly. My wedding band went sailing across the room! I had lost so much weight, my ring no longer fit my finger! The wedding band was recovered, and my marriage is still very much intact.

My first forty-day fast was more of a protest against the Vietnam war than most people realized. I really thought I was going to die! I would come back to a hotel room somewhere after giving a lecture, flop down on the bed and fall asleep. Then I'd wake up in the middle of the night and pinch myself to see if I'd died in my sleep. I'd never died before, so I began to think, "Wow! Maybe this is what death feels like! One everlasting pinch!"

So I would call Dr. Fulton in Chicago, and she would reassure me. More important, she would tell me *exactly* what was going to happen on each day of the fast! When Dr. Fulton told me that at the end of the third week of fasting I would feel a resurgence of energy like I had never felt before, well, I won't say I *dis*believed her; I'll just say I didn't believe it at the time! But of course it was true, because at that period of the fast the body begins *consuming itself,* ridding the system of stored-up poisons and waste that have been there for years.

On January 9, 1968, I broke my first fast, with fruit juice, at the Fultonia Health Food Center in Chicago. After a long fast, Dr. Fulton says, it is necessary to take a day of fruit juice for every five days you have been fasting, so I needed eight days of juice before I could begin eating again.

What began as an act of social protest—a political act—became in the process of living it a "purifying act"—in mind, body and spirit. As my body was cleansed of years of accumulated impurities, my mind and spiritual awareness were lifted to a new level. I felt closer to Mother Nature and all her children. I felt more in tune with the universal order of existence. I was now aware of the meaning of the words I used to hear in church: "The body is the temple of the spirit." Just as Jesus drove the moneychangers out of the temple, fasting had driven the "devils of my former diet" from my own "temple," and my life changed completely.

About three months after my first fast, I had a sip of Scotch and soda and the taste was repugnant. That old favorite devil of mine was gone forever. I then remembered how bad liquor tastes to most people the first time they try it. Folks say you have to "cultivate a taste" for booze. Even though the body is saying "No!" people repeat alcohol until they get used to it.

With my body cleansed from fasting, I had a new hunger. I hungered to know more about nutrition and proper food so that my "temple" would remain clean. I visited health food stores everywhere I traveled. I would head straight for the book rack and buy every book on health and nutrition I could get my hands on. I found more wisdom there than I've found on any college campus I've ever visited—and I lecture in three hundred colleges a year.

The more I read, the more I talked with Dr. Fulton and the more I experimented with my own diet, the closer I came to the fruitarian point of view concerning nutrition. After my first fast, I adopted a diet that included only raw foods. I became convinced I should leave my "cookin'" to Mother Nature!

I've fasted many times since my first forty-day fast, sometimes for health reasons and sometimes for *vocational* reasons. The longer fasts have been the results of my vocation in the struggle for human dignity.

Beginning in 1968, my vocation has involved me in a fast every summer. In the summer of 1968 I served forty-five days in the state prison in Olympia, Washington, as a result of my participation in a demonstration with the Nisqualli Indians, who were demanding their fishing rights. In the summer of 1969 I served forty-five days in Chicago's Cook County Jail as a result of leading daily demonstrations during the summer of 1965, protesting de facto segregation in the Chicago public schools. During both periods of confinement I took only distilled water for nourishment.

In 1970 I spent most of the summer in a house I had rented in Toronto, Canada. I fasted eighty-one days on distilled water. It was a "public" fast, which I announced to the news media.

I was fasting to call attention to the narcotics problem in America. I explained, in announcing my fast (which I originally intended to last forty days), that fasting cleanses the body of all impurities; that the bad food most people eat each day is flushed out; and the body is given a fresh start for a new and more healthy future. I said further that I hoped my fast would help people to recognize the poisons infecting the national body, to see the need for cleansing the nation of impurities, so that America could have a fresh start toward a new and more healthy future. Of course, I was also fully aware of the "private" benefits of fasting, so my fast had public and private reasons.

I was trying to make a personal witness to the tragedy and hypocrisy of the drug problem in America—tragic because America's youth suffer most from the deadly effects of narcotics; hypocritical because the American system allows the drug traffic to continue while berating the drug users for their affliction.

I refused to believe that a nine-year-old kid could find the Heroin Man any time he needed help in sending destruction through his young veins, yet law enforcement officials couldn't find him— the pusher, the supplier, the smuggler. I refused to believe that the same Federal Bureau of Investigation that couldn't prevent narcotics from being smuggled *into* the country seemed to have no trouble at all stopping espionage activity, keeping American security secrets from being smuggled *out* of the country.

At the time of this writing, I am on a fast which began April 24, 1971. While speaking at an outdoor rally in San Francisco, I was moved once again to make a personal witness in protest against the senseless killing in Indochina. I announced, at the end of my speech, that I would not eat any solid food until the war is *over* in Vietnam. I have been on a liquid diet ever since, taking fresh fruit juice for nourishment.

Perhaps a cleansing fast is needed by the American peace negotiators to see the truth about the war from a clean, pure perspective. I wonder how many bogged-down negotiations have taken place over lunch and dinner? If eating hasn't ended the slaughter, fasting should be worth a try. But the American way of life still favors the consumption of both meals and countries. The country has moral, as well as physical, constipation.

When the war is finally over, I shall maintain a fruitarian diet. Which means I've traveled most of the way along the Continuum of Consumption. I don't know if I'll ever reach the final breatha-tarian stage completely, though I have had limited encounters with this plane of living over the past summer (1972).

At the end of August and into the early part of September, I went on two seven-day total fasts—no food, no water, no solid or liquid nourishment of any kind. My diet consisted only of air, sunlight, bathing in pure water, and frequent enemas with water warmed by the direct light of the sun. My first seven-day total fast took place in Jalapa, Mexico, while I was staying at the Hotel Lagunita. I was accompanied by my close friend Adam D. Bour-geois, a Chicago attorney and veteran faster, who also completed the seven-day total fast.

Ten days later I went on another seven-day total fast at the Milk River Mineral Baths on the beautiful island of Jamaica. The Milk River Baths are among the unsung miracles of Mother Na-ture, the water there being as therapeutic as any in the world. I hope some readers of these pages will do themselves a great favor and visit Milk River.

As you can see from my nutritional autobiography, I started out in life poor, with almost nothing, and I ate everything. Now I have almost everything, and more often than not I choose to eat nothing. But more than any wealth or fame I have achieved, I consider my journey along the Continuum of Consumption the real success of my life. I have learned that the highest value in life is really a "family affair." It is coming home to Momma. No mat-ter how far away you may have traveled, Mother Nature is always waiting for your return!

3

On Being Fruit-Full and Multiplying

As I said in the last chapter, I come from a large family. So I guess having a lot of kids comes natural to me. My wife and I have nine kids. In fact, my wife, Lillian, had so many babies at the same hospital in Chicago, they put a revolving door on her room in the maternity ward! A few years back, some Southern white folks used to bad-mouth me for having so many kids. A friend of mine once told me that Governor Wallace of Alabama even accused me of trying to grow my own race!

I can't comment from personal experience upon the relationship between proper diet and fertility. Lillian and I chalked up quite a record of fruitfulness before we became full of fruit. And with all the family planning enthusiasts telling us the family of the future should have no more than two and a half kids, the less I say about fertility the better. I would have to say, though, that a couple has a better chance of producing that half a kid if they are eating wrong than if they are eating right!

But it does stand to reason that life should spring most naturally from life. When a couple feeds upon Mother Nature's living diet, fruit and vegetables, they should have a better chance of bringing *new life* into the world than if they are feeding themselves upon death—the cooked flesh of animals that have been killed.

I have seven girls and two boys. My cast of children, in order of appearance, is Michele, Lynne, Pamela and Paula, my twins, Stephanie, Gregory, Miss, Christian, and the newest member of the cast, Ayanna. I beg your indulgence of a proud father as he comments on some of the names. The twins, Pamela and Paula, have the middle names Inte and Gration, which of course combine to form the word "integration." The twins' middle names will be a reminder throughout their lives that during the period of her pregnancy, their mother was jailed in Selma, Alabama, while demonstrating for freedom, justice and the cause of human dignity in an integrated society.

My oldest son, Gregory, has just one name. His birth certificate does not read "Gregory Gregory," but rather simply "Gregory." In the American system, whose computers, bureaucracy and institutional requirements *demand* two names to function, my son Gregory is a symbol of independence of the built-in entanglements which predetermine the destiny of the "two-namers" in a controlled society.

Gregory's younger sister, on the other hand, has two names. She is Miss Gregory. At the time of her birth, racial hangups in the United States made it difficult for some white folks to call a black woman "Miss" and a black man "Mister." So to be on the safe side, my wife and I named our daughter Miss. All her life, anyone who calls her by her proper name will have to say, "Miss Gregory."

My youngest daughter has the African name Ayanna, which means "beautiful flower." She is the child closest to Mother Nature from birth, having been conceived and born during the most advanced period of her parents' nutritional awareness and appreciation of the natural way of life. As a true child of Mother Nature, she shares kinship with a beautiful flower.

Earlier this year, 1972, I got my second wife. Don't get me wrong. I didn't remarry! My marriage bond with Lillian has not been broken. But I have a *new* Lillian. Lillian began the year with a diet of three months of fruit juice, after which she went on forty days of only water. Her weight dropped from 200 to 140 pounds, and her dress size diminished from 22½ to 14!

But, in all honesty, I would have to say I am Lillian's third husband. When we were married, I was on the slender side. Then I ballooned up to the 280-plus figure described in the last chapter. And now I am below 100 pounds, much less than my weight when we were married. I guess we're one of the few couples who can claim a second wife and a third husband and never have engaged in bigamy, polygamy or divorce!

Although my whole family is now on the same diet, some of the kids have shared the dietary transitions of their parents. Four of the girls were in the family while I was still a carnivore. (I also had a son, Richard Claxton Gregory, Jr., who died in 1962 at the age of two and a half months.) The twins, however, were just a little over a year old when I became a vegetarian, so they hadn't had a chance yet to be heavy into meat-eating.

I am often asked if I get a lot of family resistance when I make a dietary change in the household. Over the years, I have developed a system for making those changes which seems to work very well. I pick certain key times in the year, like when school closes for the summer or opens again in the fall or the first of the new year, and announce to the family in advance when a certain dietary change will take place. I have found it helpful for the kids to be given a chance to prepare for a change in their eating habits rather than having it sprung on them suddenly. This method is called benevolent dictatorship.

The first big change in the family diet was the elimination of meat from the menu. But I didn't drop *all* meat from the diet overnight. I did it over a six-month period, which might be a helpful pattern for anyone who wants to become a vegetarian. For the first three months the family menu included only fish and chicken. After the three months had elapsed, we dropped chicken and permitted only fish for the next three months.

Next to go were candy, potato chips, salted peanuts, cookies, doughnuts and all of the other snack items one buys at the supermarket or candy store. At the same time we dropped white bread, replacing it with brown bread, and white refined sugar, which was replaced first with brown sugar and then with honey. There were no racial overtones in dropping all that white stuff from the diet. It was merely the conviction that the so-called enriched and refined products were really bleached, denatured and devitalized. You make out of *that* what you will!

Then we dropped milk, cheese and eggs. Finally, after wiping out the dairy barn and the henhouse, we stopped eating cooked foods entirely and reached the present stage of the family menu: only raw fruits and raw vegetables and their juices (after the nursing period has ended). The only dietary changes since dropping cooked foods have been with regard to seasoning—like eliminating salt and pepper in favor of more natural herb and seed seasonings.

The major change I have noticed as a parent, as new offspring come into the Gregory household and start off with proper eating habits, is the absence of the usual children's sickness. What most folks call the "normal" childhood diseases just simply do not exist for us. There are no running noses in my household, and if anyone calls one of my offspring a "snot-nose kid," it is purely metaphorical. Even the dictionary will admit that "to snivel" is "to snuff mucus up the nose audibly." And where proper eating habits eliminate excess mucus in the body, the need for sniveling is gone.

So I now have kids in my household who may never know what a medical doctor looks like, unless they just happen to bump into one on the street! Or unless they break an arm or a leg. Of course, this was not always the case. And surprisingly, it was not always the case *even after the changes in diet*! For at first after the family diet began to include more and more fruit and fruit juices, the kids began to develop rashes and other skin problems. In the winter rashes appeared where their heavy wool coats rubbed against their neck. I took them to a skin specialist, who gave them vitamin E ointment. We used the ointment, continued the same diet, and the skin problems eventually disappeared. Then I learned what had been causing the problems. It was not the diet, but rather the effects of improper eating habits *before* the change in diet. The fruits and juices were having a cleansing effect on the system, and the stored-up poisons and mucus were being eliminated from the body and coming out through the pores.

I remember an experience we had with Pamela, one of the twins. Some time after her diet had been changed, a knot appeared on her arm about the size of an egg. I thought it was rather strange that eggs removed from her diet would appear on her arm! So I took her to Dr. Roland J. Sidney of Chicago, our family naprapath. (A naprapath is a doctor of the natural healing arts.)

Dr. Sidney massaged Pamela's arm during a series of treatments, and all of a sudden, one day the "egg" disappeared. Dr. Sidney explained that the knot on her arm was collected mucus which had settled in that particular spot. When she was a baby, Pamela had a chest condition, with a great amount of mucus in her chest.

When her diet changed, the mucus began breaking down and draining out, and for some reason it settled in the one spot on her arm.

My experience is an important lesson for anyone who begins to follow a natural diet. You can expect to have problems. The degree of difficulty will depend on how bad your diet has been before. The stored-up poisons and waste in the system will start coming out and you are bound to feel the effects—rashes, or headaches, or whatever. But don't be alarmed. If you hadn't changed your diet, you would probably not have felt the effects for a few more years. Then the poisonous by-products of improper eating might have hit you all at once in the form of cancer, arthritis, cirrhosis, or some other major, catastrophic ailment.

When the quite natural, normal physical manifestations of a system being cleaned out appear, go to a naprapath or chiropractor for treatment. They will work with Mother Nature rather than against her. They will be able to provide natural, nonchemical treatment: massages, realignments, adjustments and other ways of assisting Mother Nature's natural processes.

Or you can provide home treatment. When swelling appears, massage the area gently and often. Also dilute the fruit and vegetable juices consumed by adding pure water to them. Above all, do not stop the natural diet. Do not become alarmed that something in the diet is causing physical disorders. The diet is causing the body to regain health and it must first undo the damage done by earlier eating habits.

There's a great fringe benefit of eating a natural diet and it is a shame more poor folks don't realize it. The absence of sickness means no doctor bills. From my experience in life, I would say most poor folks spend about a third of their time and earnings treating illnesses—caring for sick members of the family, pay-ing doctor bills and hospital expenses, buying medicines. And of course they are the folks who can least afford such a toll.

I have often said poor folks should eat more like rich folks and rich folks should eat more like poor folks. I would not advocate that anyone eat the wrong kind of food, but if anyone *does* it should be the wealthy, because they can afford the medical expenses which are sure to follow bad eating.

In reality, eating habits are just the opposite. The rich eat well (as society defines this) and the poor eat poorly. Rich carnivores can afford the choicest, freshest meats. They can afford the luxury of garden-fresh vegetables and orchard-fresh fruits. Many rich folks have their own gardens and orchards. It is also interesting to note that the homes of the wealthiest families have a tendency to be located in truck farming areas, giving the rich immediate access to freshly grown and freshly cultivated crops.

Poor folks, on the other hand, take their food stamps or their meager earnings to the supermarket. They buy canned foods, frozen foods, TV dinners, white bread, pastries and all other kinds of commercially processed junk. The meats, vegetables and fruits in the supermarkets in poor communities are always of the lowest quality and are sold at the highest prices! The result is that poor folks pay more to eat their way into even greater expenses.

Mothers and fathers in poor communities work so hard to earn money to feed their families, and they have such a difficult time making ends meet. The real tragedy is that they do not realize it is cheaper to feed those families correctly than it is to purchase the junk diet. For example, the prices of meat, milk and eggs are always skyrocketing. Each time there is a price hike, it hurts the poor more than anyone else. Yet meat, milk and eggs are all items poor folks—and all other folks—would be better off not eating!

Let me close with a few parent-to-parent words.

Raising kids is such a chore these days. You're supposed to learn how to reason with them and communicate with them rather than punishing them as in the old days. It was a lot different when I was a kid. I remember when my daddy wanted to punish me, he'd just say, "Get on upstairs to your room." Which was a terrible punishment, because there *wasn't* any upstairs!

I remember one time I told my daddy, "Dad, if you don't give me a nickel, I'm gonna run away from home!" He didn't even blink as he said, "I'm not giving you one single penny—and take your brothers with you!"

To show you how different things are now, not long ago my daughter Lynne announced, "Dad, I'm running away from home. Call me a cab."

I said, "Lynne, honey, you don't know how lucky you are. When I was your age, my family was poor, we never had enough to eat, rats and roaches in the house, no heat or hot water in the winter—" Lynne broke in and said, "Dad, aren't you glad you're living with us now?"

Kids are so sophisticated these days. I just found out the other day you don't walk into a kid's room anymore. You have to knock first!

And hip! I found out how really hip kids are a number of years ago on Christmas Eve. I went into my oldest daughter's room and told Michele to go to sleep before Santa Claus came. She said, "Dad, I don't believe in Santa Claus." I exclaimed, "What do you mean, you don't believe in Santa Claus?" And she shot back, "Because you know darn good and well no white man's gonna be in our neighborhood past midnight!"

When you make changes in your own family menu, be prepared to have some very energetic kids on your hands. The energy level of my children is higher than ever before. They sleep well when they should be sleeping. They are very alert and extremely active when they should be up and enjoying life to its fullest.

Be prepared also to face the problem of others trying to impose wrong eating habits on your children. So many folks will feel sorry for your kids because they are not allowed to eat the things so-called normal kids eat. Remember, it is your kids who should feel sorry for the others' eating habits. If a snack is served in school, you must inform school officials of your children's diet and send over the food your kids are to eat (if the school cannot satisfactorily provide it).

I have found it necessary to cut out party attendance for my kids almost entirely. They only go to birthday parties and the like at the homes of very close friends. My close friends understand that my children will take their own food with them. If the kids stop by a friend's home after school, the parents are informed they are to be served absolutely nothing. I don't trust juices served away from home, as they are usually canned or frozen, and I don't even want my kids drinking tap water if I can help it.

Don't be shocked, surprised or alarmed at your kid's change in appearance. When you start following the natural diet, there will frequently be weight loss, especially in the face. Parents sometimes become worried because they associate chubbiness with health. That theory is only the rationalization of an ill-fed America.

Finally, in a family where the diet is wholesome and natural, and the family members enjoy increased health, vitality, energy and mental capacity, there is also more love in the home. There is more love present because the true momma of us all has taken up residence. When Mother Nature comes to live in your home or apartment, the whole family shares the blessings and feels the vibrations of her maternal love like the warm glow of the rays of her morning sun.

4

The Body Owner's Manual

Most folks go through life as though they truly believed the opening words of that old song: "I ain't got no *body!*" The average person has no idea of the *location* of the organs, glands, vessels, nerves, arteries and other components of the body, to say nothing of a lack of knowledge of their *function.* And that internal ignorance is probably the best explanation for the kind of "food" most people shove into their bodies.

It is characteristic of the American dream for folks to work very hard to earn enough money or credit to surround themselves with pieces of machinery—a television set, a refrigerator, a dishwasher, a stereo, a clothes washer and dryer, and of course an automobile. But before they've earned a penny, Mother Nature has provided them with the finest mechanism imaginable—their own body. Yet most people appreciate this marvelous piece of equipment the least.

The tragic truth is that most folks treat their automobiles better than their own bodies. If it was definitely proved that smoking cigarettes in an automobile would instantly corrode the engine, every smoker would quit smoking in his car! No automobile owner would pour refined sugar into the gas tank, or stuff a steak in the carburetor, or shove wet, soggy white bread into the radiator. Automobile owners would refrain from such things because they know it would damage their precious machines.

Also, automobile owners are constantly in search of the best possible fuel for their cars. They are careful to change the oil regularly and see that the car is periodically lubricated. They check the owner's manual provided by the manufacturer of their car to see that they are treating their machine correctly. Yet the car owner will park his automobile, run into a luncheonette and wreak havoc upon his personal machine!

This chapter is intended to serve as a brief Body Owner's Manual for the care, keeping and understanding of that marvelous machine Mother Nature has given to us free of charge. Although everyone will one day have to face that "final recall" of the body machine, the length and quality of service depend upon how well the operational demands of the mechanism are understood and the care it is given.

The Filtering System

There are a number of glands in the body engaged in the filtering process, but the two major filters are the liver and the kidneys. In a car owner's manual, you are advised to change the filter periodically. Medical doctors sometimes offer the same advice for the body machine, calling the process of changing filters "transplants." While it is good, in fact essential, to cleanse them through proper diet, Mother Nature's filters usually carry a lifetime guarantee if treated properly.

THE LIVER

Everything we eat or drink is broken down and carried by the blood to the liver. In the liver, the atoms and molecules of our food are reconstructed into material which the body uses to repair, replenish and rebuild cells and tissues.

Thus the liver is certainly one of the most important and amazing glandular organs in the entire body machine. It is the largest gland, making up about one-fortieth of a person's total weight. And the liver has miraculous powers of regenerating and healing itself. Which, of course, is a blessing to most people, considering the punishment they inflict upon the liver through improper diet. If heart or brain cells are damaged and die, they cannot be replaced. But the liver, given the nourishment needed to heal itself, can remarkably "come back to life." Most abused livers need only a decent opportunity for "personal resurrection."

The liver performs a number of complex chemical functions in the body. Rearranged molecules and atoms are sent back into the bloodstream from the liver and are distributed to the other glands and parts of the body as they are needed. The by-products of the reconstruction work in the liver, along with used-up cells from other parts of the body system, are converted by the liver into bile. The bile is collected and stored in the gall bladder and is used as needed in the digestive process and other functions of the body.

The liver is burdened with the work load of undoing the damage inflicted upon the body by improper eating and drinking habits. Poisons and narcotics which would destroy the body if left alone are passed as quickly as possible to the liver. The liver cells neutralize the poisonous components and try to convert them into harmless chemical compounds. It's as though the rest of the body were saying to the liver, "Dig, baby, see what you can do about what this fool just ate and drank!"

When raw fruits and vegetables and their juices are consumed, the liver performs its functions normally. Only raw, live, vital organic food has the magnetism needed to aid in the bodily functions. So when cooked or processed foods are consumed, foods which have lost their vital natural magnetism through the application of heat, the liver has a big job on its hands. The liver has to try to reconstruct inorganic, lifeless atoms and molecules. Starches, grains, meat products and anything that has been cooked in fat give the liver a tremendous workout. Starch molecules, for example, when passing through the liver, can become lodged in the liver cells. When this happens often enough, a congestion develops which can result in cirrhosis or hardening of the liver. The liver becomes stiff as a board. The diet prepared in most kitchens may be responsible for that common phrase "room and board."

It is interesting to note that most people think of cirrhosis of the liver as a disease peculiar to heavy drinkers. While it is true that heavy drinkers are inviting this disaster, it is also quite possible for a heavy starch consumer, or a big sandwich eater, to develop cirrhosis without having had a drink of alcohol during an entire lifetime. Concentrated protein, such as meat, is also difficult for the liver to handle, and eating it runs the danger of clogging liver cells and causing inflammation. The liver has to work double duty trying to deal with fat that has been cooked to as little as 96 degrees Fahrenheit. And no matter how "lean" meat is, there is always some fat.

Let me offer an example, suggested by N. W. Walker in his excellent book *Become Younger*, to illustrate what most folks do to their liver every day. If a person bought a truck, and the owner's manual said the load capacity was a half ton, the new truck owner would be a fool to load up the truck with two or three tons and run it day in and day out. The truck would carry the load for a while. But one day it would break down and the owner would be running to the bank for a loan on a new truck. It's the same with the load capacity of the liver. Most folks overload its capacity every single day of their lives, three meals a day. And the liver handles its burdened load for a time. One day it is likely to break down.

Before the truck breaks down completely, it will slow up, the tires will give way, the springs will sag and the frame will be pushed out of shape. And the overloaded liver will bring about the same reaction in the human body. Consider the person suffering from a "sluggish" liver—slow, lifeless movements, feet lagging, and frequently a bent frame!

THE KIDNEYS

The other major filters are the kidneys—two glandular organs about the size of a human fist, suspended by a ligament from the rear wall of the abdomen. Hanging loosely near the spinal column, the kidneys serve the function of filtering the water in the body as it is passed through them by the bloodstream.

The kidneys are another of Mother Nature's miracles. They are made up of more than thirty billion cells grouped into clusters of miles and miles of little filter coils. Each cluster is no larger than a speck of dust, yet contains some fifteen thousand cells. These tiny coils filter four gallons of water every day. Only two to four pints are passed as waste through the bladder and eliminated as urine. The remaining water is recirculated by the bloodstream throughout the body system.

Every drop of liquid consumed is filtered through the kidneys. The blood is about three-fifths water, and that water content remains constant no matter how much is taken in. Excess water taken in above the three quarts in the blood is stored in the muscles and the liver. But it is all filtered by the kidneys.

Everyone knows what happens to water that is left standing and is not replenished by a flow of fresh, pure water. It becomes stagnant. The same thing happens in the body. It is very important to replenish the body with pure drinking water or the organic water which comes from raw fruit and vegetable juices. Pure water in the body system is the most important element in proper maintenance, with the exception of oxygen in the air.

Transmission Fluid

The **bloodstream** is the transmitter of food throughout the body system and at the same time the garbage collector. There are about four quarts of blood in constant circulation out of the six quarts or more in the body machine.

To appreciate the marvel of the circulating bloodstream, it might help to realize that your blood deals in more billions than the United States Department of Defense! The bloodstream is composed of some twenty-four or twenty-five billion microscopic cells. They travel so fast through the body machine, it would make the astronauts' and the NASA engineers' heads swim. Every fifteen to twenty-five seconds, the twenty billion-plus cells travel the whole route, from head to foot, through the heart and to the lungs to get a fresh supply of oxygen and leave behind the carbonic-acid gas from the body system. Those twenty billion-plus cells make from three thousand to five thousand round trips through the body machine every twenty-four hours!

So every second of the day and night, billions of blood cells are traveling through the heart and into the breathing chambers of the lungs. And each and every one must have proper nourishment for the journey. The next time you're tempted to make a diet of pastries and coffee, stop and think if your blood cells will find it ideal fuel for the distances they must travel. And think of the work load of the blood cells in a mere sixteen cupfuls of blood.

Every cell and tissue of the body is constantly being bathed in **lymph fluid**. The lymph is a fluid substance made up of cells known as lymph cells; white blood cells or corpuscles, or leuko-cytes; and scavenger cells known as phagocytes. So completely is the body machine covered with lymph vessels for the bathing and lubricating process that if the lymph vessels were placed end to end in a straight line they would span a distance of over 100,000 miles.

The lines of the intestine, for example, are filled with lymph nodes, or knots, which continuously serve as security agents in the body to guard against the intrusion of destructive substances and liquids. Millions of other lymph security guards are located at strategic points in the body machine. For example, a specially refined lymph (cerebrospinal fluid) cushions the brain and the spinal cord against the walls of bone surrounding them. The con-dition of this lymph is very important in maintaining the mental and physical balance of the body machine.

Such seemingly simple acts as standing up, walking, running and other physical movements are completely dependent upon the healthy functioning and the balanced relationship of the brain and the spinal cord. The muscles receive their impulses for phys-ical movement from the spinal cord and the coordination comes from the brain. The ear channels are also filled with lymph. Every time the head is moved one way or the other, the lymph level changes. You can't agree or disagree without the lymph being in-volved! Thus the lymph is very important in keeping the physical equilibrium of the entire body machine.

The transmission fluid, the blood and the lymph, and the transmission system, the lymph and blood vessels, must be kept clean and free of clogging. Clogging, or capillary impactions, can result in such things as defective hearing, dizziness, eye trouble, unsteadiness, hemorrhoids, varicose veins, hardening of the arteries, tumors and blood clots on the brain or elsewhere in the body machine. Starches of all kinds, fried foods and other cooked fats are the great cloggers.

When functioning according to Mother Nature's design, the lymph nodes in the intestine collect fats, but they do not collect protein or carbohydrate material passing through. The collected fats are converted into a fine liquid, or emulsion, and passed into the main lymph channel in the throat and then on into the bloodstream. Mother Nature's system works very smoothly when the fats are raw, uncooked and natural, such as in olive oil, avocado, raw nuts, and so on.

But if you throw fried foods, buttered popcorn, cooked salted nuts or doughnuts at the lymph security agents, try as they will, they may not be able to break down the fat, since it has been converted by cooking into an inorganic product, and the fat may remain in circulation in the blood for hours, resulting in a clogging of the system. So that popcorn you eat in the movie theater may be creating a late late show in the body machine!

One further word about starches. The body machine takes the "fuel" provided by the owner and breaks it down into atoms and molecules—the smallest particles into which matter can be broken down. For example, the formula for water, as almost everyone knows, is H_2O. The smallest particle of water is composed of two atoms of hydrogen and one atom of oxygen. The formula for the starch molecule is $C_6H_{10}O_6$—six atoms of carbon, ten atoms of hydrogen and six atoms of oxygen.

The starch molecule is not soluble in water, alcohol or ether. Heavy consumers of white bread, breakfast cereals and other starchy foods are inviting all the ailments accompanying clogging. Starch eaters shouldn't be surprised to develop deposits of gravel and stones in the kidneys and the gall bladder.

Since the starch molecule travels around the body machine in an undissolved state, unable to be used by the glands, cells and tissues of the body, the body machine tries to flush it out. If the organs designed to take care of eliminating waste become clogged, the body machine looks for other places to throw the starches out. The pores of the skin provide a perfect opening. And Mother Nature provides even for her most disobedient children. Germs thrive on starchy matter and they assist in breaking down accumulated starch molecules, forming pus, which is more easily pushed out through the pores of the skin. Instant pimples! Teenagers with acne and pimple problems will probably be found to have heavy starch diets.

The Carburetor

The **lungs** are made up of tiny bunches of cells similar to grapes, microscopic in size and about 400 million in number. The importance of the lungs is emphasized by the fact that the body machine can operate days, weeks and months without food; at least days and perhaps weeks without water; but only a few minutes without air. The blood cells and corpuscles must have oxygen to burn up waste matter, break down the structure of food and liquid, and make available atoms and molecules to the cells, tissues and glands of the body machine.

The machine takes in about a pint of air at a time, or 20,000 pints a day, or 2,500 gallons. After each intake of air, the body lets out millions of molecules in the form of carbonic-acid gas. That's the in and out performance of the body machine according to Mother Nature's ideal design, with no interference in the carburetor.

When foods are eaten which produce a high degree of mucus

in the system, such as cow's milk and starchy foods, the excess mucus lodges in the lungs (as well as other places in the body). The little bunches in the lungs become so tightly clogged that oxygen can't get through. The same thing happens, of course, when cigarette smoke or polluted air is inhaled. This is in addition to the nicotine content of cigarettes, which has an extremely poisonous effect upon the system.

When debris settles in the lungs, shutting off the flow of a fresh intake of oxygen, Mother Nature's body machine tries to compensate. It steals oxygen from the carbonic-acid gas (CO_2) which is supposed to be expelled. When the oxygen is thus "borrowed" from CO_2, CO, or carbon monoxide, is left in the system. Carbon monoxide is known for its deadly effect. People who want to end it all go into the garage, close the doors, turn on the engine of the car and breathe in the carbon monoxide fumes from the exhaust pipe. Others, of course, choose the slower method of suicide by a lifetime of "relaxation" through cigarette smoking.

Incidentally, the "relaxing" or "soothing" effect upon the nerves cigarette smokers claim to rationalize their habit is really nothing other than a deadening or anesthetizing of the nerve centers. Death is indeed ultimate relaxation!

The Fuel Pump, Battery, Spark Plugs and Other Parts

The **heart** is the fuel pump of the body machine, pumping oxygen through the bloodstream to various parts of the body according to their need. Since the heart is a living tissue, it must receive nourishment from the food taken into the body. However, it does not receive nourishment from the blood pumped through it, but rather from a special supply of blood coming through the coronary arteries.

The pumping action of the heart causes it to "beat," giving rise to the familiar political comment in the United States that the vice-president is only a "heartbeat" away from the presidency. The phrase really means that as long as the president's heart is beating, the vice-president is still away from the presidency!

The heart beats about 100,000 to 150,000 times a day, pumping somewhere between 10,000 and 11,000 quarts of blood throughout the body. Circulating the blood around at such a pace, the heart will pump some 45 million gallons of blood in the span of a half century. Few other fuel pumps could render that kind of service.

The rate of the heart, or the intensity of its work, depends upon the demand put upon it by other parts of the body. When an organ is called upon to do more work, it needs a greater supply of oxygen and thus the heart must work harder too. Exercising requires more oxygen, and the heart must pump it. So does eating. When the process of digestion is going on, glands and organs need greater supplies of oxygen from the heart. If the diet consists of the wrong kind of food, overloading the work of the liver and other parts of the body, the heart also feels the strain.

The action of the heart speeds up when the carbonic-acid gas content of the blood is increased. Eating an excess of carbon foods increases the carbonic-acid gas content of the blood and consequently "puts a hurtin'" on the heart. Starchy foods, cereals and all kinds of manufactured sugar have this effect. Too much carbon food intake results in both high and low blood pressure. It is tragically amusing to hear folks talk about "having heart trouble," when, if they analyzed their diet, they would have to admit they are "giving themselves heart trouble."

The storage battery of the body machine is the **nerve system**. During sleep the "battery system" stores up energy to replace the vital life forces. The main distributing nerve center of the body machine is located at the base of the brain in the medulla oblongata, just above the nape of the neck. There are two main divisions of the battery system: the sympathetic nervous system and the central nervous system.

The sympathetic nervous system has nothing to do with a person's sympathies but rather controls the directing force coming from the brain. Breathing, the regulation of temperature and water in the body, the organs involved in eating and drinking, regulating the distribution of blood—all these functions (and many more) are affected by the sympathetic nervous system.

The central nervous system is Operation Central in the body machine. It is the network of nerves from the brain down the spinal cord, spreading throughout the body to the skin. Operation Central sends out an alarm when anything is wrong, or out of line, in the body machine. A headache, or a toothache, or any other pain, is an alarm from Operation Central, the central nervous system. And of course the purpose of the alarm is to see that the *source* and *cause* of the pain are treated.

So what treatment do most body owners give? They take an aspirin or some type of chemical "pain killer." The result is simply to "kill" or deaden the nerve trying to do its duty. The headache, or toothache, or whatever, will disappear but the *cause* will remain unattended. It is exactly the same as the ancient custom of killing the messenger because he brought bad news to the emperor!

Every organ, limb and part of the body machine has three major nerve endings. One is in the iris of the eye. One is in the walls of the colon. One is in the sole of the feet. It is standard practice of the trained naprapath to be able to look at the eyes, the soles of the feet or an X ray of the colon and tell exactly which parts of the body machine are in trouble.

For example, the nerve at the lowest portion of the ascending colon corresponds to the pituitary gland, the gland of mental and physical balance. Persons who experience mental or physical unbalance, or epileptic fits, have been reported to have a nest of worms thriving in the uneliminated waste matter in the colon, which is causing the difficulty. If not worms, it is at least a large amount of accumulated waste matter which has piled up over the years and not been flushed out, causing severe inflammation of the colon.

When the body machine is functioning as Mother Nature intended, the nerves and the **muscles** have a good working relationship. The nerves send out the impulses and the muscles get to work. They are such a team that if something is done to mess up one teammate, the other is usually directly affected.

Meat is an enemy of the muscles, which in turn makes it a potential foe of the nerves. Meat is bad for the muscles because it tempts them so. Muscles have a particular attraction to uric acid, the end product of the digestion and breaking down of protein molecules. Uric acid should be expelled through the kidneys. But because of the muscles' attraction to it, they absorb the uric acid before it can be eliminated, especially when there is an excess.

Finally the saturation point is reached. The uric acid begins to crystallize in the muscles. When the crystal-containing muscles are moved, the sharp points penetrate the covering of the nearest nerve and a sharper pain is registered. It's the first warning of later trouble—rheumatism, neuritis or sciatica. Heavy meat-eaters often have *seven* to *twelve* times as much uric acid *retained* in their system as should have been eliminated through the kidneys in the first place.

Gas and the Body Machine

There is a very old joke about the roadside restaurant that had fuel pumps out front to serve the needs of passing motorists. The sign read: EAT HERE AND GET GAS. And that sign pretty well sums up the traditional American diet!

Of course, the "gas" we're talking about here is not the kind you'll find in a car owner's manual. We're talking about the natural chemical action in the body machine whereby matter is converted from a solid or a liquid into a gaseous state.

After food has passed through the stomach and the small intestine, bacteria in the body machine go to work on the residue of food as part of Mother Nature's design. The function of the friendly, helpful bacteria is to break down the residue so it can be absorbed for constructive purposes. It enters the colon from the small intestine as a liquid. The ascending colon goes to work on the liquid, taking out most of the water and the food elements the body machine will use, and sends the remaining fibrous substance on to the next sections of the colon as feces to be eliminated.

The domelike portion of the upper stomach collects the gas which develops as a result of this digestive process. And when raw natural foods are eaten, the small quantity of gas released through the work of the digestive juices can be handled quite well by the stomach.

When foods are eaten haphazardly and in the wrong combinations, like meat and potatoes, bread and butter and perhaps jam, fruit and sugar, ice cream, pie or cake, coffee and sugar, the incompatible mixtures cause a great deal of fermentation. Belching is a consequence of the consumption of canned, cooked and processed foods.

The "dead" fibers in cooked foods hinder the work of the entire intestinal tract. While the fibers in raw foods *assist* the work of the intestines, the habit of eating cooked dead food causes the intestinal walls to lose their tone and degenerate over a period of time. Waste matter is not properly eliminated, and it adheres to the walls of the intestines, accumulating in the pockets of the colon.

The result is a regular gunfight or shootout in the body machine between the "good" bacteria and the "bad" bacteria. The "good" bacteria try to neutralize the waste matter and eliminate it. The "bad" bacteria find it very comfortable living quarters and try to get the waste matter to remain. The result of the "shootout" is an excessive amount of gas. The average restaurant meal, beginning with cocktails (alcohol is very gas-forming) and ending with coffee and sugar, is a regular "showdown at the OK Corral."

Although a certain amount of gas in the intestines is natural and inevitable, excessive gas can cause a host of ailments, including what frequently passes for a heart attack! Gas pressure against the heart and blood vessels can send a person scampering for digitalis tablets when an enema would be more in order.

The Sewage System

This is probably the most important section of the Body Owner's Manual. It has been claimed that nine-tenths of the physical disorders and diseases of body owners have their origin in the **stomach** and **intestines**. The two great abuses body owners inflict upon the machine Mother Nature has given them are the failure to *nourish* the organs in the body responsible for the proper elimination of waste matter and the failure to give *careful* and *immediate* attention to Mother Nature's call that waste matter must be eliminated.

First, let us trace the route of food as it leaves the plate. Food is chewed by the **teeth**, manipulated by the **lips**, **tongue** and **cheeks**, and moistened and softened by **saliva** fluid. The saliva also has a chemical action on the food, and it begins the digestive process. When food is gulped or chewed very little, the digestive process is thrown out of balance from the very beginning.

To digress for a moment, not long ago the macrobiotic diet began to enjoy wide popularity, especially among young people. All of a sudden reports were heard of macrobiotic diet enthusiasts suffering from malnutrition and physical disorders. Without going into the macrobiotic diet thoroughly, the major neglect of those who followed the diet was the failure to chew the food properly—hundreds of times for each bite.

Food which has been chewed and insalivated in the mouth reaches the stomach through a drainpipe called the **esophagus**, entering at the upper opening of the stomach. Then the stomach begins its own process of digestion by secreting a fluid called the **gastric juice**. The gastric juice begins to dissolve and break down the mass of food so that it can be absorbed into the body. While this chemical action is going on, the fluid portion of the food and the liquids which have been consumed are being separated from the solids, absorbed through the walls of the stomach and taken by the blood to the kidneys, the skin pores, and so on. The stomach muscles are busy churning up the digested food and creating a semifluid food mass of chemically changed matter which passes into the **small intestine**.

The small intestine is about an inch and a half in diameter, some thirty feet long, and ingeniously wound around upon itself so that it occupies only a small place in the body machine compared to its length. The entire length of the small intestine is lined with a soft velvety covering of tiny little projections known as villi.

The wall is also lined with millions of glands that secrete enzymes needed for the digestion of various food elements.

In the small intestine the digestive process of breaking down food elements is completed. The enzymes secreted from the walls of the small intestine are assisted by enzymes secreted by the pancreas and bile provided by the liver. When the breakdown is completed, the digested food element is ready for absorption into the lymph system. It is picked up by the villi, which contain blood and lymph vessels.

Food that *cannot* be digested because of its nature, or *is* not digested for some other reason, is left behind in the form of waste matter, excrement, feces or any of the more popular names. It is dumped into the large intestine, or **colon**, eventually to be eliminated from the body machine. The waste matter passes into the colon through a small opening known as the ileocecal valve. The valve is constructed to let the waste matter pass freely into the colon but to prevent it from getting back into the small intestine.

There are a number of reasons why food reaches the colon undigested or only partly digested. Sometimes it is not chewed well enough. Sometimes too much food has been eaten and the digestive system just couldn't handle it all. Or an imbalance or insufficient supply of digestive juices might interfere with proper digestion. And, finally, foods that are eaten together in improper combinations can greatly overtax the digestive system and end up in the colon undigested.

The colon is about six feet long and it connects with the small intestine on the lower right side of the abdomen. It extends upward until it reaches the lower ribs, crosses over to the left side and then heads downward again. The portion on the right side going up is called the **ascending colon**. The portion crossing over from right to left is called the **transverse colon**. And the portion going

down on the left side is called the **descending colon**. The point
where the colon and the small intestine meet is called the **cecum**.
And the other end of the colon, from which the waste matter is
expelled, is called the **rectum**.

The colon is the great sewer of the body machine. What happens to waste matter when it reaches the colon is very, very important to the health of the entire body. When the waste matter gets
to the colon, billions of bacteria invade the vegetable foods and
help to disintegrate them. The undigested or partly digested part
of protein—especially meat protein—undergoes putrefaction. As
it putrefies in the colon, it releases some very toxic by-products.
If these toxins are not neutralized and rendered harmless by the
liver, or counteracted by other bacteria in the colon, they can
cause great damage throughout the body.

The walls of the colon contain tiny absorbent channels which
have a tendency to reabsorb the foul, putrefying, poisonous excrement back into the system. If the colon becomes clogged and
if proper elimination does not take place, the whole body is poi-
soned. In fact, this retention of poison in the body is the root
cause of all disease. Poisonous toxins retained in the body produce
a condition of toxemia. And the way to begin restoring health to
the body according to Mother Nature's design is to take steps to
detoxify, or unpoison, the body. It is done through fasting and by
following a diet of raw, natural foods and juices.

The habit of eating cooked foods is the greatest ally toxemia
has. A person who eats mostly cooked foods cannot possibly have
an efficient and healthy colon, even though bowel movements
may occur two or three times daily. We tend to think of constipation as no bowel movements. And certainly that is one sure way to
know waste matter is piling up in the body machine. If food is going in and nothing is coming out, something is backed up some-

where. But if we think of constipation as *improper elimination*, or incomplete elimination, daily regularity has nothing to do with it.

Only the fibers of raw fruits and vegetables furnish nourishment to the nerves, muscles, cells and tissues of the walls of the colon. Their bulk is needed in the colon just as it is needed in the small intestine. The fibers of raw foods assist in creating the gentle, wavelike contractions in the colon known as peristalsis, which is necessary for the proper elimination of waste matter. The waste matter is propelled along by the process of peristalsis on its way to the rectum and out of the body.

Cooked foods actually starve the colon, and though a starved colon may let a lot of fecal matter through, it is anything but healthy. Cooked, devitalized foods passing through the colon leave a coating of slime on the walls like plaster on the walls of a house. Over a number of years, the coating of fecal matter becomes so impacted on the colon walls that there is only a very small hole through which the waste matter can pass. The impacted colon becomes inflamed and distorted and the collected waste matter remains in the body, sending toxic poisons throughout the entire system.

The colon may become so filled with accumulated waste matter in an adult that it stretches to a circumference of fifteen inches! Obviously the increased weight of the colon displaces it in the body machine. A heavily impacted colon may fall down into the pelvis. Also, the colon may become so full that it presses against other organs located in the abdomen, interfering with their functioning. The colon may press against the liver and interfere with the flow of bile, or against the urinary organs and interfere with the elimination of urine.

If this discussion of the effects of a clogged colon sounds a bit disturbing, it is only because it should! If a body owner becomes disturbed enough about the condition of the colon now, a great deal of trouble can be avoided later in life. And what can the concerned body owner do?

Let me answer by asking another question. What would you do with any other clogged sewer? You would flush it out, of course. You would get some Drano or Instant Plumber, or call Roto-Rooter, and go to work. Remember the colon acts just like your drain at home. When the toilet or the sink becomes clogged, all of the collected waste material backs up, and if something is not done quickly it spills over. In the same manner, a clogged colon spills toxic collected waste into the entire system.

If you have a clogged personal sewer, you have a lot of company. Reports from hospital autopsies indicate that only about a tenth of the patients have anything like normal colons. Almost everyone carries around five to ten pounds of deeply buried toxic poisons. Some of the symptoms are familiar to most folks—sour stomach, indigestion, heartburn, headaches, a weary, run-down feeling, bad breath, pimples, nervousness, feverishness, dry skin, yellow eyeballs, to name but a few.

If the idea of taking enemas turns you off, think of "internal baths" as a solution. When the outside of your body machine gets dirty, you give it a bath. So if the *inside* of your body is "dirty," why not give *it* a bath? Let me add a further word for the enema paranoids who may be reading these pages. I said in the beginning that this is a book about my own personal experience—what I have learned in my new life of "cookin' with Mother Nature." And one of the most important lessons is the necessity of keeping the colon as *clean* and *well-flushed* as possible.

The term "colonic irrigation" may be unfamiliar to most readers. It is, to use a dictionary-type definition, "the application of a continuous stream of water into the colon for the purpose of cleansing, disinfecting, etc." A colonic irrigation requires the use of an irrigating machine and a trained operator. It is not a home remedy.

If you are interested in a colonic irrigation, find a naprapath or chiropractor. He will probably be able to tell you where a colonic is available. If there is a health food store in your community, you can ask there.

There are many different kinds of colonic irrigating systems. The essential requirement is the expertise of the operator, who must be someone trained in anatomy and particularly familiar with irregularities of the colon. It is helpful for the operator to have an X ray of the patient's colon to give a key to the most effective type of treatment. A good colonic irrigation takes from three-quarters of an hour to an hour. The number of colonics required depends, of course, on the condition of the patient's colon. A series may be necessary.

The home remedy for treating a clogged colon is the "high" enema, and it is the only "high" I recommend! (Drug, tobacco, alcohol and coffee "highs" have no place in my natural diet.) An enema bag is available from any drugstore. It is a "hot water bottle" equipped with a syringe, a long tube with a nozzle. This enema equipment is different from prepared and packaged enemas, so be sure to ask for an enema bag. A prepared enema will clean out only the lower part of the descending colon rather than give the entire colon a flushing.

The standard enema bag will hold about two quarts of water. It should be suspended from the wall at least three feet above you. Most supermarkets sell suction hooks which can be fastened to the bathroom wall, moved to any other wall or carried when traveling.

The water used for an enema should be lukewarm. Never, never use soap, salt, bicarbonate of soda or any other such substance in the water! It is helpful to add the strained juice of freshly squeezed lemon—one, two or even three lemons for two quarts of water—and a teaspoon or two of pure unpasteurized honey. But never add anything else.

Some authorities have recommended three or even four quarts (one gallon) to cleanse the colon; but two is adequate and causes less discomfort. It may be necessary to start with one quart and work up to two.

The object is to get the water well into all parts of the colon. Some people prefer a kneeling position. Others prefer to lie on the right side, with the legs doubled up toward the chest as in a fetal position. The nozzle of the syringe should be lubricated with K-Y surgical jelly. The water should be retained in the colon as long as possible.

Especially in the beginning, some discomfort may be felt. Don't be alarmed or discouraged. After a while, the feeling of discomfort will ease and more and more water will be able to be retained in the colon. As in all other new ventures, practice makes perfect in enema-taking.

Massage the abdomen gently while retaining the enema water to help loosen the impacted waste matter. Don't be surprised to find yourself hurrying back to the bathroom. I only mention it to warn you that it is not best to run off to any business or social engagements too soon after taking an enema!

After the flushing is over, you may notice that you pass more water than usual from the kidneys. This means that some of the water has reached the kidneys from the colon by absorption. It is good for the kidneys to have a beneficial flushing.

The time set aside for flushing the colon is up to the individual. Some prefer the evening just before going to bed. Others prefer the morning. For a thorough initial colon flushing, it would be good to take a dozen enemas on the following schedule: three days in succession, three days every other night, three days every third night; then three times more once a week.

Laxatives, cathartics, purgatives, and the like are a different matter. A laxative does not help to restore the natural process of peristalsis in the colon. On the contrary, the laxative is actually an irritant. That's what makes a laxative a laxative. It irritates the nerves and muscles in the colon, sending them into a state of convulsions to get rid of the irritating substance. The laxative, or purgative, challenges Mother Nature rather than working along with her. It in no way helps to break down impacted waste matter or cleanse the colon. Taking a laxative is like throwing salt in the eye to produce tears to wash out a cinder!

Some people refuse to take enemas because they believe it will become habit-forming. It is much easier to develop a laxative habit than an enema habit. But an internal bath should be no more habit-forming than an external bath.

Actually, the best way to assist Mother Nature in the process of elimination in the body machine is through nutrition. The *very* best way to help Mother Nature is to *drink a glass of warm water containing the juice of one freshly squeezed lemon every morning immediately upon arising.* You'll be amazed at the results.

The Headlights

The headlights of the body machine are the eyes. Using another analogy, the eyes are the windows to the temple. One can quickly tell the condition of the body machine by looking at the headlights. If they are dim, dull or the color of fog lights, the body machine is in bad shape and in drastic need of immediate repair.

The fuel must be changed. A diet must be provided which allows for a complete rebuilding job.

If the eyes are shiny, sparkling and bright, it is an encouraging sign that the body machine is close to kicking on all cylinders. So as a conscientious body owner, take a good look in the mirror and see if the headlights in your own machine are on bright or dim.

Let me close this chapter with a vision and a hope for America. The Body Owner's Manual clearly suggests that the body machine is worth at least as much attention as an automobile. What is needed in this country is as many health food stores as there are filling stations and auto repair shops. Each health station should be staffed with folks who are as well versed and trained in nutrition and the proper care of the body as good mechanics are in the care and keeping of automobiles.

Wouldn't it be wonderful if all the rest areas along the turnpikes and superhighways of this nation were both service stations *and* health food stores and restaurants? Now that would *really* be a trip!

5

Food or Somethin' to Eat?

There is a difference between *food* and *something to eat*. Just as there is a difference between *diet* and *nutrition*. Most folks would define "diet" as "the food that is eaten." And they would go on to say that a "good diet" equals "good health."

I'd like us to be a little more precise in our common journey along the Continuum of Consumption. *Diet* is the *food that is consumed*. That's right so far. But *nutrition* is the *food that is consumed that the cells and tissues of the body can utilize*. And that is a most important addition. You can have a very large diet in terms of food consumed and be literally starving your body in terms of nutrition.

So now you might think the proper formula should read: good diet plus good nutrition equals good health. That's pretty close, but still not quite right. The correct formula would be: good nutrition plus good assimilation equals good health. Of course, if someone rates "good" on the nutrition consumption it follows that such a person's diet will also be good.

Having agreed upon a working formula, let's establish why we eat—or rather what should be the *real* reasons why we eat. We all know most folks determine the items in their diet by taste alone—we eat something because it tastes good. But the real reasons why we eat should be: to gain new cells and rebuild the various body tissues; to get starch to heat our bodies, the necessary oil to lubricate the machinery of our bodies, and fibrous matter to keep our tubing clean; and to make our tissues pliable to provide a means of circulation for our blood corpuscles. In short, to keep our body machine in good working order.

It must be admitted that all this is not easy to do with the type of junk that passes for food in the average supermarket. The American diet explains, perhaps, why more than eighty nations of the world have a lower death rate than we do in the United States. A hundred or even fifty years ago, your grandparents or parents had an easier time relating to Mother Nature. Their water was pure and unpolluted. When they inhaled deeply, they were not taking in carbon monoxide fumes. Their food was grown organically, often in their own gardens. The soil was well manured and the fruits and vegetables had no residues of poisonous sprays, waxes and chemical treatments. Eggs came from healthy chickens eating worms, bugs and natural grains. The wheat for bread contained as high as 24 percent of protein. Candies, soft drinks and canned foods were luxuries for the rich, and processed foods were all but unknown.

But today eggs are usually laid by chickens who never see the light of the sun and eat chemically treated mash. Much so-called enriched white bread has lost more than forty vital nutritional elements, including vitamin E, and in turn has been loaded up with chemicals. Our depleted soil is hyped up with chemical fertilizers; many meat and dairy products are permeated with DDT, preservatives, hormones, and drugs and chemicals.

To relate to Mother Nature today requires a real effort. You're better off at a health food store, but if the supermarket is your only recourse, you can find something to eat although you'll be pushing your shopping cart past most of the shelves!

The Dick Gregory Shopping List

Walk on by the frozen food counter. That means no TV dinners, or frozen fruits and vegetables. These are not quick-frozen foods but rather processed foods with preservatives added and other various and sundry chemical treatments. Let me give you a simple example. Take frozen French fried potatoes. If you have ever peeled a fresh potato, you will know that the potato turns brown wherever you touch it in the process of peeling. Yet the potatoes you see in the freezing compartment are peeled, sliced and whiter than the average suburb. Have you ever thought why? Because the potatoes are treated and bleached to give them the snow-white color!

Walk on by the canned foods also. They too have been heated and treated, thus destroying all of the most important life-giving elements. That's how I know Popeye is a fraud. He's always eating *canned* spinach. There's no way he could get anything other than an impacted colon from that diet! If he was munching on raw spinach leaves, I could believe in him.

Though it may sound strange coming from me, I advise you also to walk past the canned and bottled fruit and vegetable juices. They too have been heated and treated with preservatives. Anything that has been pasteurized must be bypassed. The pasteurizing process destroys the enzymes, which in turn renders the "food" useless to the body machine. So bypass pasteurized vinegar and honey. Only pure apple cider vinegar and pure unrefined honey should be purchased.

Speaking of processed juices, one of my favorite examples is frozen orange juice. It is obvious that additives are placed in frozen orange juice. How many times have you read in the newspaper that citrus farmers in California or Florida feared that an unexpected drop in temperature would ruin their crop of oranges? Heating pots are placed strategically in the orchards in case of such emergencies, and when the temperature drops to freezing, the pots are lighted in an effort to save the crops. If that's what freezing does to oranges, doesn't frozen orange juice seem rather suspect to you?

Continue on, bypassing the breakfast food shelf. Breakfast cereals are completely devitalized. But don't be discouraged—*some* things in the cereal line are for you. A good general rule to follow in shopping is "Caveat emptor," or "Let the buyer beware." Unfortunately that is still the attitude in America rather than the more moral position, "Let the seller be honest!" You will arrive eventually at the fruit and vegetable counter, the nut and seed rack. Among these nuts, fruits, etc., is everything necessary for your diet, with the single exception of pure water. The chief constituents in good nutrition and assimilation are proteins (or more accurately amino acids), carbohydrates (sugars and starches), fats, and minerals and vitamins. And they are all available here. When using your fruits and vegetables, be suspicious of chemicals and sprays and use the disinfecting process described in Chapter Nine.

You might want to carry in your wallet or purse a shopping list which includes the minerals in order of their importance and suggests the foods which supply them. The list is taken from pages 33–34 of N. W. Walker's *Diet and Salad Suggestions*, slightly modified to exclude all animal products.

Calcium: Unsalted almonds, carrots, dandelions, turnips, spinach, oranges, okra, cauliflower, tomatoes, garlic, parsnips, all berries, all nuts (except peanuts and cashews), apples, potatoes, apricots.

Phosphorus: Kale, large white radishes, asparagus, sorrel, watercress, Brussels sprouts, garlic, savoy cabbage, carrots, cauliflower, squash, cucumbers, leeks, lettuce, turnips, Brazil nuts, walnuts, huckleberries, blackberries, cherries, black mission figs, oranges, limes.

Potassium: Carrots, celery, parsley, spinach, beets, cauliflower, leeks, garlic, potatoes, sorrel, squash, tomatoes, turnips, oranges, lemons, apricots, bananas, cherries, dates, grapes, huckleberries, figs, pears, peaches, plums, raspberries, watermelon, pomegranates, olives.

Sulfur: Brussels sprouts, watercress, kale, horseradish, cauliflower, cabbage, chives, garlic, sorrel, cranberries, raspberries, pineapple, currants, apples, Brazil nuts, filberts.

Sodium: Celery, carrots, spinach, tomatoes, strawberries, radishes, squash, lettuce, dandelion, leeks, cucumbers, beets, turnips, apples, apricots, watermelon, huckleberries, pears, oranges, grapefruit, lemons, dates, cherries, grapes.

Chlorine: Beets, cabbage, celery, garlic, horseradish, parsnips, sweet potatoes, tomatoes, avocados, dates, pomegranates, coconut.

Fluorine: Unsalted almonds, carrots, beet tops, turnip tops, dandelion, spinach, celery tops, cauliflower, cabbage, watercress, parsley, cucumbers.

Magnesium: Carrots, celery, cucumbers, unsalted almonds, dandelion, garlic, leeks, kale, lettuce, tomatoes, spinach, lemons, oranges, apples, blackberries, bananas, figs, pineapple, Brazil nuts, pecans, walnuts.

Iron: Lettuce, leeks, carrots, dandelion, radishes, asparagus, turnips, cucumbers, horseradish, tomatoes, almonds, avocados, strawberries, raisins, figs, watermelon, apricots, cherries, huckleberries, walnuts, Brazil nuts, apples, grapes (particularly Concord), pineapple, oranges.

Manganese: Parsley, carrots, celery, beets, cucumbers, chives, watercress, almonds, apples, apricots, walnuts.

Silicon: Cucumbers, lettuce, parsnips, asparagus tips, beet tops, dandelion, horseradish, leeks, okra, parsley, green peppers, radishes, spinach, watercress, strawberries, cherries, apricots, apples, watermelon, figs.

Iodine: Spinach, asparagus, carrots, green peppers, pineapple, okra, turnip greens, cucumbers, watermelon.

Bear in mind that all of the items on your shopping list are considered in the raw form. Take horseradish, for example. I am by all means not referring to prepared bottled horseradish, but rather to raw horseradish, which you will grind or liquefy yourself in a blender and take in half-teaspoonful quantities at a time. Nuts are uncooked and unsalted. Do rule out peanuts and cashews. Peanuts are legumes, not nuts, and they have an acid action in the body. Cashews are seeds of the cashew fruit and are hard to digest.

Other items not mentioned on the shopping list are also good for you (melons are probably best eaten alone in as large quantities as you desire). And don't forget sun-dried fruits, especially when fresh fruits are not available, but be sure you are getting dried fruits that have not been treated with sulfur. Dried fruits should be placed in a bowl, barely covered with distilled or pure water and soaked until they are soft.

If we take the same list of materials given above, but focus on the top five foods which provide each mineral, we find some new items cropping up.

Calcium: Whole sesame seeds, kelp, Irish moss, agar, dulse.

Phosphorus: Rice bran, wheat bran, pumpkin and squash seeds, wheat germ.

Potassium: Dulse, kelp, Irish moss, soybeans (dried), lima beans (dried).

Sulfur: Kale, watercress, Brussels sprouts, horseradish, cabbage.

Sodium: Kelp, Irish moss, olives, dulse, hot dried red pepper.

Chlorine: Ripe tomatoes, celery, iceberg lettuce, kelp, spinach.

Magnesium: Kelp, wheat bran, wheat germ, almonds, soybeans.

Iron: Dulse, kelp, rice bran, wheat bran, pumpkin and squash seeds.

Silicon: Lettuce, parsnip, asparagus, dandelion, rice bran.

Iodine: Kelp, dulse, agar, Swiss chard, turnip greens.

Although the lists are nearly identical in some cases, as with sulfur, there are some items on the second list which may be somewhat unfamiliar. But all of these foods are important to proper nutrition. I'm referring particularly to the seeds—sesame, pumpkin and squash (to which I would also add sunflower)—and the sea vegetation—kelp, Irish moss and dulse.

The most important item for you on the cereal shelf is wheat germ. Wheat germ is the embryo, which makes up only about 2 percent of the grain, but it is the most important percentage nutritionally. Wheat germ contains the E, B and A vitamins, and is the richest source of nourishment for the body's growth and reproduction.

Sea Hunt

Many nutritional experts believe that sea vegetation contains *all* the vitamins and *all* the minerals if used in their natural form and in combination. They excel all other sources of vitamins and minerals, natural or artificial.

Dulse is a red seaweed gathered for centuries by the Irish off their coastline. Kelp is the catchall name for a variety of large brown seaweeds abundantly available off the coast of Japan and along the west coast of the United States. Government documents have reported that oil extracted from seaweed contained one thousand times more vitamins A and D than an equal quantity of cod liver oil. Which, of course, stands to reason. The seaweed is where the cod's liver got it in the first place!

Sea plants contain not only an abundance of iodine, iron, copper, manganese and cobalt, all essential in the formation of hemoglobin, but also all of the vitamin B complex, so important to anyone suffering from anemia. One cannot help wondering why sea vegetation, like dulse and kelp, is not more universally available and why it has not replaced synthetic or artificially manufactured chemical products as "multiple vitamins." I feel the answer is simply that sea vegetation is cheap and readily available, and its use would not yield the large profits the chemical-vitamin industry demands!

It is worth a trip to the health food store just to get dulse and kelp. They're certainly a better addition to all items in your diet than table salt and it would be a good idea to get into the habit of sprinkling dulse and kelp powder on your foods. You'll be getting vitamins A, B, C and D in abundance, along with vitamin E, the antisterility vitamin, and vitamin K, which has an antihemorrhaging effect. And by all means, if you suffer from goiter trouble, run, don't walk, to the nearest health food store and get some dulse and kelp.

Seed Hunt

If you will recall some of the stories that fascinated you in your childhood days, you will no doubt remember the phrase "Open Sesame!" It was a magical incantation, and the very mention of the word "sesame" unlocked a multitude of mysteries and charms. The person who possessed sesame was the holder of many riches.

The magic word refers to the sesame seed. Its nutritional properties were held in such high esteem in the Orient that it became synonymous with magic. Sesame seeds are valuable because of their high content of calcium and phosphorus, combined with their complete protein. They contain 50 percent more protein (amino acid content) than meat. Milk made from sesame seeds (a recipe for which appears later in this book) is far superior to cow's milk for human consumption. It is further improved when combined with coconut milk.

Sesame seeds do not putrefy (or rot) in the intestines as meat does, so those who use them avoid the dangers of constipation and the toxic poisoning of the system. Sesame seeds, by the way, are a good base for an eggless mayonnaise for those who are adopting the wise practice of a no-animal-product diet. The seeds may be liquefied in a blender and combined with honey and lemon juice.

When purchasing sesame seeds, look for imported ones. Domestic sesame seeds are more likely to have been grown with chemical fertilizer than those coming from South and Central America, China and the Near East. An added benefit of sesame seeds is that they are cholesterol-free!

Pumpkin seeds and squash seeds are perhaps the tastiest of the seeds. The squash seed is a high-fat seed which is exceptionally digestible and full of nutrition. It is rich in fat-soluble vitamins and lecithin, a source of B vitamins which metabolizes fats and helps to cure fatigue and weakness, as well as skin disorders.

Until recently, most sunflower seeds in the United States were consumed by the parrot population. They were even referred to as "polly seeds." And of course it is not uncommon for a parrot to outlive its owner. The unhip parrots stood around saying, "Polly wants a cracker."

The vitamin content of sunflower seeds is exceptionally high. They have the vitamin B complex and vitamins D and E in abundance. Sunflower seeds contain three times the protein of meat and, like sesame seeds, they do not putrefy. They are also cholesterol-free. The mineral content of sunflower seeds is high, as any farmer can tell you. The sunflower plant feeds so enthusiastically on the minerals in the soil that it quickly exhausts all the available supply. These minerals are stored in the seeds. Since the roots of the sunflower plant go down deeper than those of most vegetables, sunflower seeds are a source of minerals not found in vegetables.

While I have been noticing more natural seeds and nuts in the supermarkets, it is a shame that 99.9 percent of all the items offered for consumption are processed junk. I do hope readers of these pages will raise a fuss with supermarket managers in their community and let them know that if they store pure, raw natural foods it will profit them. Drugstores should be pressured into stocking natural vitamin supplements, at least along with, if not instead of, the artificial, chemical supplements. I long to see the day when all supermarkets and drugstores become true health food stores. Then the markets would have a reason to call themselves "super"!

Coffee, Tea or Milk

You've noticed I have avoided animal products—milk, eggs, cheese and the like. I can hear some of you wondering right now: "But I always thought milk was the perfect food." It probably is—for a calf! Few human mothers would consent to nurse a calf, but they let the cow nurse their own babies. As Dr. Paul Gyorgy of the University of Pennsylvania said in the November 2, 1972, issue of *Jet*: "Human milk is for the human infant. Cow's milk is for calves." Although milk is generally praised as a calcium source, the most important ingredient is a substance called casein, which furnishes a number of amino acids for supplying the protein molecules to build bone structure that will carry the body's weight. The casein content in mother's milk is appropriate for a human baby. But in cow's milk the casein content is appropriate for building a baby calf. Cow's milk contains three hundred times more casein than mother's milk. It is intended to grow a calf into an adult weighing about three-quarters of a ton! Cow's milk is designed to double the weight of the calf in a period of six to eight weeks. A human baby requires six to seven *months* to double its weight. It is little wonder that so many babies fed on cow's milk have an excess of mucus, as in running noses, congested chests, etc.

Casein, by the way, is the material that makes the finest quality glue for woodwork. Cabinetmakers can use it more effectively than human babies. So it's probably the milk in oatmeal that sticks to your ribs.

The same indictments apply to milk as to other pasteurized products. The heating in pasteurization destroys the enzymes. It is possible to get certified raw milk and raw milk cheese at the health food store, but I would recommend its use only for household pets for reasons noted above.

The singular exception I make to the rejection of animal products is *plain* yogurt. Yogurt is rich in predigested proteins and in vitamins B_1 and B_2. It establishes an acid medium in the intestinal tract which inhibits the growth of harmful and putrefaction-causing bacteria. In other words, yogurt replaces the "good" bacteria which may have been lost in flushing out the colon.

Having disposed of milk, what about coffee and tea? Both coffee and tea are stimulants and both contain caffeine. That alone is enough for me to rule out the use of coffee and standard teas. I have read studies comparing caffeine to morphine in its destructive properties. Just as I wouldn't support the neighborhood pusher, I'll not let the grocer push coffee or commercial tea in my direction.

A small drop of caffeine injected into an animal's skin will produce death in a few minutes. A very, very small amount injected into the brain will create instant convulsions. Who knows what effect caffeine has in the coffee cup? Also, coal tar from coffee has the same dangerous characteristics as the coal tar found in tobacco. And, finally, coffee increases the flow of hydrochloric acid in the stomach. Deaths from cancer of the stomach and bladder outnumber lung cancer deaths in this country and it would *seem* that there could be a relationship to the coffee-drinking habit.

At the health food store you will find a dandelion coffee some people regard as an excellent substitute, and a great variety of herb teas: ginseng, camomile, peppermint, alfalfa, sarsaparilla, Golden Seal, flax seed, safflower and fenugreek to name a few.

Next time you're looking for somethin' to eat, try some real *food* from Mother Nature, and you'll find the food your momma offers is *really* somethin'.

6

The American Diet—
Myths and Realities

When it comes to diet and nutrition, I see an analogy in the experience of black Americans which would benefit *all* Americans. It can be summed up in the admonition, "Give up the 'process' and go 'natural.'" Let me explain. There was a day in the black community, not too very long ago, when the way to be "cool" and "hip" was to go through the painful baking process of straightening out your nappy hair. The straightened hair was called "a process."

Then along came the civil rights movement of the 1960s, and with it Dr. Martin Luther King and Malcolm X and Stokely Carmichael and H. Rap Brown, telling black folks to take pride in their blackness and be as Black and as Beautiful as Mother Nature intended them to be. All of a sudden, the "process" hair style gave way to the Afro, or "natural," hair style. Black folks gave up the "process" to go "natural."

The same advice applies to diet and nutrition. Give up that processed food and start eating natural foods. Unfortunately, most black folks decided to go "natural" in every phase of their life except diet. They still cling to that "soul food." But more on that subject later in this chapter.

Tarzan and the Apes

One of the major myths plaguing the American diet is the *protein* myth. Most folks believe it is really necessary to eat meat to get the proper amount of protein in the diet. The myth goes on to say that protein is necessary for strength. Finally it becomes twisted and distorted to come out that the *strongest* man is the heavy meat-eater—the so-called meat and potatoes man.

Let's attack this myth by a quick survey of the animal kingdom. The strongest animals in the jungle are not meat-eaters. They are vegetarians and fruitarians. They don't need meat to make them strong! What are the strongest animals in the jungle? The lion— the "king of the jungle"? No. One of the sneakiest and most brutal, maybe, but certainly not the strongest. The tiger? No. The giant of the jungle, of course, is the elephant. And what does the elephant eat? Fruit, leaves and young branches. Unless the elephant is in a zoo, where peanuts may become a substitute for a jungle diet. But not hot dogs. The elephant is a vegetarian.

Want some other examples? Few other jungle creatures want to tangle with the gorilla. And what does the gorilla eat? Fruit and succulent vegetables! The gorilla is a vegan and close to being a complete fruitarian.

Then there's the hippopotamus, another jungle giant. The hippo eats grass and herbage. And the rhinoceros, certainly not a weakling by even the lion's estimate. What does the rhinoceros eat? Leaves, twigs and general herbage and vegetation. No meat!

Examining the jungle kingdom closer, we find that even the

meat-eaters don't like to eat other meat-eaters. The lion has a preference for zebra and antelope, both herbivorous animals. The tiger loves to get its teeth into a good buffalo steak, and the buffalo prefers to munch on grass.

Human beings who eat meat tend to follow the same pattern. They make pets out of the carnivores and eat the non-meat-eating animals, like cows, pigs and chickens. Although the pig is classed as an omnivore physiologically, in a natural state pigs eat grass, roots and fallen fruits. Humans will, of course, eat bears on occasion. And bears eat small animals in addition to their diet of wild berries, fruits and honey.

If we leave the jungle and look elsewhere in the animal kingdom for strength, it's interesting to note that only vegetarian animals are used as beasts of burden—the ox, the horse and the mule. And to show you what Mother Nature's soil thinks of the meat-eating habit, only the manure of vegan animals and humans is suitable for fertilizing the growth, life and power of orchard and garden plants!

So if you should lay a pork chop in front of Tarzan and King Kong, you can bet your life only Tarzan would pick it up and eat it. And I doubt that there is any argument about who is the stronger.

Meat Is Only Number Two

Exploring the protein myth further, we must remember that protein is only *one* element in the total diet. Carbohydrates, fats, minerals and vitamins must also be supplied from the food we eat. Meat-eaters who use the protein-myth argument to rationalize their dietary habits are found to be consuming much more protein than the body needs or can use.

Even more important is the recognition that when human beings eat meat, they are really eating *secondhand* fruits, vegetables, grains, etc. The bodies of animals are built from the fruit and vegetation consumed. Though in pure form when the animal eats them, they are mixed with the poisons of the animal's body by the time the human being gets his secondhand protein meal. When we eat fish, for example, we are getting our nutrition secondhand. It would be so much better to get our nourishment from the source where the fish gets it—seaweed, especially kelp, nutritionally one of the very best foods we can eat.

When the secondhand source of protein comes from the slaughterhouse, the problem of poisons in the animal's body is greatly intensified. An animal experiences a moment of terror when it knows it is about to be killed, and there is a reaction inside its body which shoots poisons instantly throughout the entire system. Adrenaline pours into the blood and muscles of the animal. Human beings have the same reaction in moments of anger, excitement and fear. And when folks die from any of these reactions it could well be the result of too much adrenaline getting into the bloodstream and not being diluted fast enough.

The adrenal glands are little caplike organs located at the top of the kidneys. They secrete a fluid that staggers the imagination in terms of strength. When a drop of adrenaline is secreted into the bloodstream, it is diluted instantly to between one and two *billionths* of its original strength. If that is hard to conceive, look at it this way. It would be the same as a single drop of ink placed in *six million gallons* of water! Or, in this day of space travel, a NASA-type analogy might be in order. Imagine two highway markers a mile apart compared with five thousand round trips to the moon!

That's what happens just *before* the slaughtered animal's death. Immediately *after* the killing, every cell and tissue in the animal's body begins to disintegrate. Between the time of bodily death (somatic death) and the *actual* death of the cells and tissues, activity is still going on. Animal tissues continue to consume soluble food material in contact with the cells and tissues, while also continuing to produce the waste substances which would ordinarily (during life) be removed to the lungs, kidneys, etc.

If the animal were still alive, these poisons would be bathed by a pure stream of blood. When the heart ceases to beat, the cleansing process stops and the poisons which are still forming accumulate at a very rapid rate. The arteries continue to contract after death until all the blood they contain is forced on into the tissues and then into the veins. Thus, the flesh of a dead animal contains nothing but poisonous blood and venomous juices!

Now doesn't it seem reasonable that it is better to eat life than death? The firsthand protein of live, fresh, raw fruits and vegetables and nuts rather than the secondhand protein of dead, rapidly decaying flesh?

Just being surrounded by death and killing takes a terrible toll on human beings. We've all heard stories of the effects of shell shock on soldiers returning from war. Harry Benjamin reports, in his book *Commonsense Vegetarianism*, that statistics show folks who work in slaughterhouses are more prone to drunkenness and disease than folks in any other type of work. Mother Nature demands a price for engaging in such activities.

I wouldn't be at all surprised if the habit of eating meat is related to alcoholism. Meat does have the effect of shocking the system the same as drugs and alcohol. Addiction to eating improper foods is quite understandably at the base of other kinds of addiction. Even brand names of booze tend to indicate a relationship. Take Beefeater Gin, for example! Did you ever hear of "Carrot Juice Drinker's Gin"?

As I suggested in my earlier book *The Shadow That Scares Me,* if meat-consumers had to do their own slaughtering, most of them would look for other sources of protein. But meat-eaters don't have to face the awful truth of the killing and death that went into the preparation of their dinners. They get the workers at the slaughterhouse to do the killing for them. By the time the meat purchaser sees the piece of steak in the butchershop window, the blood and suffering have been washed away. Or when the meat-eater orders a steak in a restaurant, it is covered up with parsley and butter, or onions, or mushrooms, and made to look appealing to the eye. It looks so attractive the meat-eater never thinks about the suffering and misery.

There is a political analogy between the restaurants and butchershops and the slums and ghettos of this nation. If the wealthy few, the moneyed aristocracy, who are responsible for the conditions of poverty and suffering in the ghettos ever walked the misery-laden streets, they would undoubtedly have pangs of conscience and would not be able to continue to perpetrate and allow such conditions.

But they are protected from the sights, smells and sounds of the slums and ghettos, just as the meat-eaters are protected from the misery and screams of the slaughterhouse. All the wealthy aristocrats ever see is the finished product, the window dressing, the steak on the platter—Thurgood Marshall on the Supreme Court bench or Senator Edward Brooke in the United States Senate. The Senate and the Supreme Court are the restaurants and the ghetto street corner is the slaughterhouse.

The Amino Theory

The secondhand protein argument seems so obvious that it doesn't need further explanation. What we're really saying is if steaks are essential for protein, why don't cows eat them? But there is a little more to be said for the benefit of the skeptics: it is not protein as such that is important but rather the *amino acids*—the protein builders.

Protein is composed of amino acids. Amino acids are compound elements composed of carbon, hydrogen, oxygen and nitrogen atoms which, when they are combined, have the function of building or constructing protein. Two amino acids contain sulfur atoms and two others contain iodine.

The protein in the flesh of animals is built up in their bodies from the live organic atoms in the raw food they eat. As such, it is pure protein. But before a human being can utilize that protein, the body must perform its own breakdown and reconstruction operation. The body must break down the animal protein not only to the original amino acids but also to the original atoms before building up its *own* protein from the original atoms and primary acids. When the human body consumes firsthand protein, the protein-building process occurs just as it does in the bodies of animals.

Let me list the principal amino acids, their composition and the food sources they come from. The following are the principal amino acids described by N. W. Walker in his book *Diet and Salad Suggestions* on pages 57–64.

Alanine: Composed of 40% carbon, 8% hydrogen, 36% oxygen and 16% nitrogen. It is important for the healthy condition

of the skin and scalp and hair, and it also is a factor in the
healthy operation of the adrenal glands. Raw foods containing
alanine are: alfalfa, unsalted almonds, avocado, olives,
carrots, celery, dandelion, lettuce, cucumbers, turnips, green
peppers, spinach, watercress, apples, apricots, grapes, oranges,
strawberries, tomatoes.

Arginine: Composed of 41½% carbon, 8% hydrogen,
18½% oxygen and 32% nitrogen. It is important to the
muscles, the reproductive organs, and the bones, and helps
to safeguard against the formation of ulcers and cancer. Raw
foods containing arginine are: alfalfa, carrots, beets, cucumbers,
celery, lettuce, leeks, radishes, potatoes, parsnips, turnips.

Aspartic Acid: Composed of 36% carbon, 5½% hydrogen,
48% oxygen and 10½% nitrogen. It is important to the bones
and teeth, the lungs and respiratory system, and the heart
and blood. Raw foods containing aspartic acid are: lemons,
grapefruits, unsalted almonds, apples, apricots, carrots, celery,
cucumbers, parsley, pineapple, radishes, spinach, tomatoes,
turnip tops, watercress, watermelon.

Cystine: Composed of 30% carbon, 5% hydrogen,
26½% oxygen, 11½% nitrogen and 27% sulfur. Among
other things it is important to the hair and the formation
of red blood corpuscles. Raw foods containing cystine are:
alfalfa, carrots, beets, cabbage, cauliflower, chives, onions,
garlic, kale, horseradish, radishes, Brussels sprouts, apples,
currants, pineapple, raspberries, hazel nuts, filberts.

Glutamic Acid: Composed of 41% carbon, 6% hydrogen,
43½% oxygen and 9½% nitrogen. It is involved in the
secretion of digestive juices and in enzymic action in the
liver, and helps to avoid anemia. Glutamic acid is formed
by eating raw string beans and Brussels sprouts, carrots,

cabbage, celery, beet tops, turnip tops, dandelion, parsley, lettuce, spinach, papaya.

Glycine: Composed of 32% carbon, 7% hydrogen, 42½% oxygen and 18½% nitrogen. It is a factor in the formation of bones and muscles and an influence on the sex hormones. Sources of glycine are such raw foods as: carrots, dandelion, turnips, celery, parsley, spinach, alfalfa, okra, garlic, unsalted almonds, figs, oranges, lemons, huckleberries, raspberries, pomegranates, watermelon.

Histidine: Composed of 46% carbon, 6% hydrogen, 21% oxygen and 27% nitrogen. It is involved in the control of mucus in the system, among other functions. Raw foods which are a source of histidine are: horseradish, radishes, carrots, beets, celery, cucumbers, endive, leeks, garlic, onions, dandelion, turnip tops, alfalfa, spinach, apples, pineapple, pomegranate, papaya.

Hydroxyglutamic Acid: Composed of 37% carbon, 5% hydrogen, 49% oxygen and 9% nitrogen. Raw food sources of hydroxyglutamic acid are: carrots, celery, parsley, lettuce, spinach, tomatoes, grapes, huckleberries, raspberries, plums.

Hydroxyproline: Composed of 46% carbon, 7% hydrogen, 36½% oxygen and 10½% nitrogen. It is particularly important to the work of the liver and gall bladder. Raw food sources of hydroxyproline include: carrots, beets, lettuce, dandelion, turnips, cucumbers, almonds, coconut, avocado, olives, apricots, cherries, figs, raisins, grapes (particularly Concord), oranges, pineapple.

Iodogorgoic Acid: Composed of 25% carbon, 2% hydrogen, 11% oxygen, 3% nitrogen and 59% iodine. It is involved in all glandular functions of the body. Note the list of good sources of iodogorgoic acid and see where fish get their firsthand supply: dulse, kelp, sea lettuce, carrots, celery, lettuce, spinach, tomatoes, pineapple.

Isoleucine: Composed of 55% carbon, 10% hydrogen, 24% oxygen and 11% nitrogen. It is important to glandular activity during growth, and also helps regulate general metabolism and regenerate red blood corpuscles. Raw food sources of isoleucine are: all nuts (*except* peanuts, cashews and chestnuts), avocado, olives, ripe papaya, coconut, sunflower seeds.

Leucine: Same composition as isoleucine. It has a counter-balancing effect on isoleucine and yet the sources in raw foods are the same.

Lysine: Composed of 49% carbon, 10% hydrogen, 22% oxygen and 19% nitrogen. It is involved in the actions of the liver and gall bladder. Raw food sources of lysine are: carrots, beets, cucumbers, celery, parsley, spinach, dandelion, turnip tops, papaya, alfalfa, soybean shoots, apples, apricots, pears, grapes.

Methionine: Composed of 40% carbon, 7½% hydrogen, 21% oxygen, 9% nitrogen and 22% sulfur. It is involved in the functions of the spleen, the pancreas and the lymph glands. Some raw food sources of methionine are: Brussels sprouts, cabbage, cauliflower, sorrel, kale, horseradish, chives, garlic, watercress, pineapple, apples, filberts.

Norleucine: Composition and sources are like the rest of the leucine group.

Phenylalanine: Composed of 65½% carbon, 7% hydrogen, 19% oxygen and 8½% nitrogen. It is important in the elimination of waste matter from the system. But when booze is consumed (that's alcohol), phenylalanine loses most of its effectiveness. Some raw food sources are: carrots, beets, cucumbers, spinach, parsley, tomatoes, apples, pineapple.

Proline: Composed of 52% carbon, 8% hydrogen, 28% oxygen and 12% nitrogen. It helps in the breaking down of fats in the system, among other things. Raw food sources of proline include: carrots, beets, lettuce, dandelion, turnips, cucumbers, almonds, coconut, avocado, olives, apricots, cherries, figs, raisins, grapes, oranges, pineapple.

Serine: Composed of 34% carbon, 7% hydrogen, 46% oxygen and 13% nitrogen. It helps in cleaning tissues. But smokers wipe out its effectiveness, since it is inefficient in the presence of nicotine. Some raw food sources of serine elements are: horseradish, radishes, leeks, garlic, onions, carrots, beets, celery, cucumbers, parsley, spinach, cabbage, alfalfa, papaya, apples, pineapple.

Threonine: Composed of 48% carbon, 9% hydrogen, 24% oxygen and 19% nitrogen. It helps in the exchange of amino acid atoms in the body, and the raw food sources include: ripe papaya, carrots, alfalfa, green leafy vegetables.

Thyroxine: Composed of 23% carbon, 1½% hydrogen, 8% oxygen, 2% nitrogen and 65½% iodine. It is involved in many glandular activities. Raw food sources of thyroxine include: dulse, kelp, sea lettuce, carrots, lettuce, spinach, turnips, tomatoes, pineapple.

Tryptophan: Composed of 65% carbon, 6% hydrogen, 15% oxygen and 14% nitrogen. It is involved in the functions of the gastric juices and the generation of cells and tissues. Raw foods which help to maintain the tryptophan balance include: carrots, beets, celery, endive, dandelion, fennel, string beans, Brussels sprouts, chives, spinach, alfalfa, turnips.

Tyrosine: Composed of 59½% carbon, 6% hydrogen, 26½% oxygen and 8% nitrogen. It is important to hair coloring, cell and tissue building and various glandular activities. Raw food sources of tyrosine include: alfalfa, carrots, beets, cucumbers, lettuce, dandelion, parsnips, asparagus tips, leeks, parsley, green peppers, spinach, watercress, almonds, strawberries, apricots, cherries, apples, figs, watermelon.

Valine: Composed of 51% carbon, 9½% hydrogen, 27½% oxygen and 12% nitrogen. It also is involved in glandular activities. Valine elements are available from such raw foods as: carrots, turnips, dandelion, almonds, lettuce, parsnips, squash, celery, beets, parsley, okra, tomatoes, apples, pomegranates.

These are the essential building blocks for the construction of protein in the body. The list of foods given as sources for the amino acids is by no means exhaustive. But it gives a good idea of the kinds of foods which should be eaten and which will provide ample protein production power. Look over the list and do like the animals do—get your protein and amino acids from the fresh raw foods. By the way, the listing of amino acid sources may seem somewhat repetitious. But it is purposely so to illustrate the importance of foods that keep cropping up again and again on the list—like carrots, celery and cucumber, for example.

By now the protein myth should be pretty well dissolved. Meat is unnecessary as a source of protein, and it is harmful to the body because of its highly putrefactive character. As the Body Owner's Manual has indicated, the process of breaking down meat protein in the body generates a vast amount of uric acid, saturating the muscles, and bringing on rheumatism, etc., as well as wreaking havoc on the liver.

You Deserve a Break Today—Skip the Sandwich

The sandwich is undoubtedly America's favorite lunch item. It's thrown together with a bowl of soup for kids who come home from school for lunch. It's packed in the lunch pail or brown paper bag of kids, husbands and working women who take their noon meal with them. The busy executive will "grab a quick sandwich" when the pressures of work prohibit a more leisurely noon meal. And all along the highways and roadsides of America hamburger stands and truck stops offer ever new combinations of sandwiches. But in spite of their popularity, sandwiches are probably the worst "foods" a person can eat.

The sandwich is the world's worst violator of any natural and sane principles of proper food combinations. What happens when we eat a sandwich? When the first bite is taken, the ultrasensitive nerve endings on the tongue send a message to the brain to relay throughout the system what juices to prepare to break down the food tumbling down the esophagus.

If it is a single item of food, the brain has no trouble. If it is two items, say bread and butter, the tongue sends up two messages. The brain might have a tendency to say, "Wait a minute now, not so fast!"

What do you suppose is the reaction when one bite contains bread, mayonnaise, butter, ketchup, mustard, pickle, hamburger, tomato, lettuce, salt, pepper, and maybe a gulp of soda to send the bite on its way? The brain becomes totally confused and doesn't relay any messages at all. The proper digestive functions are not set in motion. The food is sent through the system and into the colon in an undigested state. It remains fermenting in the distillery of the colon, eventually finding its way back into the bloodstream without being digested. Only two substances enter the bloodstream directly—alcohol and honey. But of course they do so with entirely different effects. Alcohol enters to terrorize the liver and honey enters to help the whole body.

We have seen in the Body Owner's Manual what clogging and liver-destroying effects undissolved and undigested food can have in the bloodstream. And on top of all this, the "quick sandwich" is usually gulped rather than chewed, so that it is not even insalivated when it zooms down the esophagus!

Of course, the same thing happens when you mix foods in your mouth during a meal. It doesn't have to be a sandwich. Corn bread, greens and a bite of pork chop in the same mouthful will have the same effect. That is why it is important, if you have many items of food on your plate, to eat them one at a time. Some health authorities advocate the *mono-feeding system*—that is, not mixing foods at all and having only a single item at a particular meal. While this system seems extreme, it is definitely true that the practice of concocting dishes to please the palate rather than to help the digesting processes of the body has done great harm to health.

The nutritional science of properly combining foods becomes quite complex. But there are some guidelines which are helpful to anyone concerned about diet and helping the body function properly. First of all, some foods are acid-forming and some foods are acid-binding, or alkaline. The latter are sometimes called base-forming foods. The acid-binding foods should always be predominant in the diet, at about a four-to-one ratio.

Thus, vegetables and fruits, including tropical and semitropical fruits, should constitute the major part of the diet since they are acid-binding or alkaline foods. It may sound strange to some people who think fruits are acid-forming because of their taste. Remember we are not talking about *taste* but rather about the effect within the body. Fruits are acid-binding in their effect. Acidity is *not* caused by acid fruits as is commonly thought. The best thing a person who is suffering from acidity can do is eat all the citrus fruit he or she can.

The acid-forming foods are cereals of all kinds, concentrated sweets, legumes (beans, lentils, peas, peanuts and cashews), nuts and, of course, all animal products: meat, fish, cottage cheese, eggs, and the like.

Anything with seeds in it is a fruit. This means that some items commonly referred to as vegetables are really fruits—cucumbers, bell peppers, tomatoes, eggplants. Bananas are hard to classify, though some authorities put them in the legume category. And if they are placed in that category they move from acid-binding to acid-forming.

I think the confusion arises from the habit most people have of eating bananas before they are thoroughly ripened. You must wait until Chiquita Banana becomes completely "colored"! When the banana turns very brown—which is when most folks and store keepers throw them away—it is ready for consumption. And then it is a fruit, because its starch content has been converted to sugar.

I personally do not recommend eating fruits and vegetables together. You will notice that in my Natural Diet menu suggestions, which follow in Chapter Nine, vegetable salads do not include cucumbers or tomatoes with lettuce and celery and other vegetables. My own recommendation is that you should wait at least a half hour, preferably longer, between fruit and vegetable consumption. Fruits are so good, why not eat them at complete fruit meals? Fruits require very little digestion in the mouth and stomach and are quickly sent to the intestines. To eat them with equal portions of vegetables, or to eat them with vegetables at all, is to have them waiting in the stomach while the longer digestive process for the vegetables is completed.

The Hot Meal

Having talked a bit about food mixing, let's talk about the myth of the hot meal: "You need something hot to stick to your ribs!" As we've seen from the Body Owner's Manual, cooked food is more likely to be sticking to your colon!

It is hard to say how the practice of cooking food got started. A story is told that in the early stages of human development, a fire destroyed a hut in which a pig was trapped. When the smoke settled, the folks found the charred remains of the pig, tasted the flesh and found the taste pleasing. But it was another few thousand years before anyone realized it was possible to have roast pork without burning down a hut in the process!

It is quite obvious that Mother Nature has provided fire for her children's use. Saint Francis of Assisi used to say, "Brother Fire is very merry!" But there is no real reason to believe that fire has any other purpose than to provide heat.

Many experts feel that cooking had its origins in the desire to preserve food. Primitive human beings may have discovered that they could keep foods for longer periods after having cooked it, and also that they could consume certain foods that they would not have been able to eat raw because of their spoiled condition. However cooking got started, it has become entrenched in the American, and worldwide, dietary pattern. Vegetables are boiled, fruits are fried and baked, nuts are roasted and salted—anything, it seems, to "kill" Mother Nature's fresh, living raw foods. But in Mother Nature's plan *nothing* should be cooked that can be eaten raw, in its natural state.

The greatest argument against cooking is that heating any food above the temperature of 120 degrees Fahrenheit destroys the enzymes. The word "enzyme" is taken from the Greek and it is literally translated "to leaven" or "in ferment." The dictionary definition is "Any of a class of complex organic substances that cause chemical transformation of material in plants and animals." In very simple terms, we might say that enzymes are the "sparks of life." Every living thing on the face of the earth contains or is motivated by enzymes. We have already been introduced to the activity of enzymes in the body machine in the Body Owner's Manual. Enzymes control the chemical reactions by which food is digested, absorbed and metabolized. They control the release of energy for every form of physical and mental activity.

Like proteins, enzymes are produced in the body. When the body machine is functioning normally and when it is supplied with the proper raw materials in our diet, enzymes are manufactured. But when the body loses that capacity for producing enzymes, they must be supplied from vital foods in the diet. Just as enzymes are destroyed by heat in cooking, we die when our body temperature reaches 106 or 107 because the enzymes are damaged. Heat inactivates enzymes. We cannot possibly obtain living active enzymes from cooked foods.

Not only enzymes but the fibrous or woody element in food is completely lost in cooking. It is what gives shape and substance to the fruit or vegetable. Mother Nature does not intend it to be absorbed into the walls of the colon, but rather to pass through like a broom and sweep the colon clean. When vegetables are cooked, this sweeping is impossible.

It is interesting to note that animals living upon raw natural foods live to be from five to seven times the age it takes them to develop. Human beings, most of whom have a tendency to live on cooked foods, do very well if they live three times as long as it takes them to develop.

There is an organ in the human body to handle every element found in food "cooked" by Mother Nature. And wherever you go in Mother Nature's world you will find the raw food "cooked" by her sunlight is the same. But the food "cooked" by human hands varies with each kitchen you enter. And each country you visit!

Soul Food or Soil Food?

I promised earlier in this chapter to return to the subject of "soul food." Soul food has its origin in the rural South and it was the diet of Blacks during the period of slavery. It seems to have survived the period of Reconstruction in a way political power for black folks did not. And with the current emphasis upon Black Pride, soul food and soul food restaurants are enjoying renewed popularity all over the country.

The soul food diet is heavy on pork and cooked vegetables. It relies heavily on the so-called lowly parts of the animal, those meat items rejected from the tables of slave owners and masters. And the vegetable items are illustrative of the slaves' inbred African tradition of "living off the land."

Slavery and the rise of the "grand" style of plantation life in the seventeenth century created the soul food menu which survives to this day. The white folks feasted on Virginia hams, fried chicken and the richer items—at least they thought they were feasting. Slaves were issued a peck of corn and three or four pounds of salt pork or bacon each week. The pork went with what the resourceful slaves, drawing upon their inbred African tradition, could grow or gather from the land around their huts. Some of the "luckier" slaves were permitted to grow vegetables on their own and sometimes even raise some animals.

Some slaves trapped 'coons or 'possums and either stole or cajoled corn and chickens from the white folks. Of course, poor folks have a tendency to eat alike. Captain John Smith's men in Virginia found some 'possum while out searching through the trees for persimmons. Everybody loved the discovery and officers and underlings alike ate 'possum. It was only with the development of the plantation elite that 'possum would be looked upon as food for slaves and "white trash."

It was the same with cutting up the hog. The so-called best portions—ham and the best cuts of bacon, now called Canadian bacon, chops and roasts—were all fare for the mansion dinner table. To this day the phrase "eating high on the hog" survives, referring to the choice meats which are found on top of the hog.

Moving down lower in cutting up the hog, the highest of the low cuts are spareribs and flank bacon. Then there are those cuts the white folks didn't want: the entrails (chitterlings), the feet and head (snout and jowls), the stomach lining (hog maws) and neck (scrapple). A private joke among slaves was how they were able to take so many of these "leavings" and make delicacies. And there are many tales told of a master sneaking tastes from a jar of pickled pigs' feet left within his reach.

So the soul food diet helped black folks to survive during their years of hardship in America, through slavery and through the depression. But there are a few interesting observations to be made. First, during slavery the vegetables grown or gathered were organic. Slaves didn't have all the pesticides and chemical sprays which infect the vegetables used for soul food menus today. Secondly, meat was not the predominant item on the menu during slavery or the depression. Meat was a luxury. When I was a kid, there was always a pot of vegetables brewing. But meat was a Sunday luxury, a very special dietary item. At other times, meat was merely a seasoning for the pot of vegetables.

Finally, during slavery and the origins of the soul food diet, the work schedule was more strenuous. There was never a question of getting enough exercise. Master saw to that! So, many of the hazards of today's soul food consumption were avoided. The slaves couldn't load up on chitterlings, greens, yams, ribs and maws and then fall asleep on the couch watching the Monday night football game on television!

Look around the black community and you will quickly see the effects of the soul food diet. Count the bloated stomachs, the bald heads, the varicose veins, the swollen ankles. Listen to the complaints of high blood pressure, heart trouble, nervous tension, etc. All these are the result of heavy starch consumption, cooked food and greasy fried food consumption, and sugar and salt consumption. One might say folks with all those difficulties are suffering from consumption!

The November 2, 1972, issue of *Jet* magazine ran an article under the heading "Medic Links Soul Food with High Blood Pressure." A leading black heart specialist, Dr. Elijah Saunders, chief cardiologist at Provident Hospital in Baltimore, indicated that soul food might be good to you but not necessarily good for you. Comparative studies in the Baltimore area revealed more than twice as many instances of high blood pressure for blacks between the ages of thirty and sixty-four than for whites. Said Dr. Saunders: "I'm not saying don't eat soul food. We don't know enough about its relationship to high blood pressure. I am saying that if you're Black, you should limit the amount of highly-salted soul foods in your diet."

I personally would say that the quickest way to wipe out a

group of people is to put them on a soul food diet. One of the tragedies is that the very folks in the black community who are most sophisticated in terms of the political realities in this country are nonetheless advocates of "soul food." They will lay down a heavy rap on genocide in America with regard to black folks, then walk into a soul food restaurant and help the genocide along.

7

Fasting: Mother Nature's Mr. Clean

As Chapter Two explains, I am a veteran faster by now. I am familiar with all the reactions people have toward fasting, but there is one thing I never really get used to. The "eaters" keep asking such stupid questions. Every time I go on a long fast, folks are always asking me, "How do you feel going this long without eating?" And do you know, when I say, "Hungry," they act *surprised?*

Just the other day a newspaper reporter came up to me and asked, "Dick Gregory, you've gone well over a year without eating any solid food. Can you describe to me how it feels?" (He was eating a corned beef sandwich at the time.)

So I told him, "The best way I can describe it to you is by an example. Do you remember the story in the Bible, where Jesus is out in the countryside speaking to a multitude of people? And at dinnertime he performs a miracle and feeds all of them with five loaves and three fish? Well, as hungry as I am, if I had been there that day I'd have blown his whole act! Jesus would have looked down at me and said, 'Verily I say unto you, I can't believe you ate the whole thing!'"

When you go on a long fast, your friends really think you are going to die. They don't say anything, but they start treating you differently. Like, they don't loan you money anymore. I had to go to my bank to get a loan during this last fast. The man at the bank said, "Sure, Mr. Gregory, as long as you have ten cosigners who are eating."

I was visiting a friend after a year and a half of not eating any solid food. We were sitting in the living room and I fell asleep on his couch. He almost went out of his mind—especially considering the fact that I have a habit of sleeping with my eyes open!

But I have a lot of fun during a fast. One of the things that keep me going is every morning I open the newspaper and turn to the obituary column—just to look over the list of "eaters" who checked out the day before! Every time I read a list of deaths I think to myself, "I'll bet every one of them was eatin'."

I went into the men's room in an airline terminal not long ago and sat down on the toilet. Would you believe some weird cat followed me into the men's room? He stood outside the booth and shouted, "Dick Gregory?" I said, "Yeah, it's me." He said, "I thought you weren't eating." And I said, "I'm not." Now he thought he had me trapped. "Then what are you doing sitting on the toilet?" And I answered, "I'm rehearsin'." Besides, I get some of my best thinking done sitting on the toilet. So I still do it, even when I'm on a long fast.

I get two kinds of reactions from people when I'm on a fast. Some folks are really worried about me. I was down in the ghetto during a long fast and a street corner cat recognized me and came running up saying, "Dick Gregory, my man! Man, you got to eat somethin'. If you don't eat you gonna die!" And the cat was eating a swordfish sandwich, dipped in cranberry sauce and cyclamate.

Sometimes I get hate mail during a fast. One of the most interesting hate letters I ever got was during my first forty-day fast. I used to always get hate mail saying, "You nigger this and you nigger that." But about the thirty-fifth day of my first fast I received a letter which began: "Dear Mr. Gregory: This is just to remind you what I had for dinner last night—fried chicken with gravy." When I saw that I suspected that there was a black cat somewhere who hates me, 'cause I know white folks eat a lot of chicken; I *also* know who eats it with gravy! The letter went on: "Mashed potatoes smothered with butter." Well, that could be either black or white. But then the letter really gave it away: "Blackeye peas with grilled onions. Jell-O topped with whipped cream—and chilled Napoleon brandy." Napoleon brandy and black-eyed peas? There was a sick black cat somewhere in America after eating that meal!

When you're on a fast, people always remind you about eating. I was sitting on a plane not long ago next to one of those "militant eaters"—you know, the kind that attacks his plate of food. He was sitting there eating his lunch and reading a *Playboy* magazine. When he got to the centerfold, he jabbed me in the ribs and showed me the picture of the nude model. He said, "Any time you see something like that, what does it make you want to do?" I told him, "Brother, as hungry as I am, I'd put an apron on her and tell her to get me something to eat!"

Any of you readers who think that sex is the number one drive for the human being, just give up eating for about twenty or thirty days. It's been over a year and a half since I had anything solid to eat and let me tell you, an old, scroungy, beat-up turnip would make a fool out of a carload of women!

I guess one thing that helps me through the ordeal of fasting is the fact that my wife can't cook anyway. My wife's cooking is so bad that during the first week of my first fast I *gained* ten pounds! But when you go on a long fast, you've got to psych yourself out. You've got to realize you will go through some changes. You *will* get hungry. And you *will* lose a lot of weight. I've lost so much weight and had my trousers taken in so many times that the right pocket is where the left-hand side used to be and vice versa.

So you have to make certain little readjustments. For example, you can't be disturbed about having to buy your clothes in the children's department. Of course, it is kind of annoying when they lay those balloons and lollipops on you! My wife said to me the other day, "If you lose any more weight, what are you going to do for underwear?" I told her, "That's easy. Lipton tea bags!"

Of course, this last fast I've been on has been longer than I had expected. I did hope the war in Vietnam would be over before the time of this writing. A television reporter asked me the other day, "Mr. Gregory, with the type of commitment you have, if the war in Vietnam ends and another war breaks out, would you give up eating again in protest?"

I answered, "No way, baby. I wouldn't give up eating again if they were fighting outside my house!"

Let me put it this way. If Rhodesia attacked Harlem, I wouldn't stop eating to protest the war. Now don't get me wrong. I'm always going to protest war and killing. If another war breaks out after the war in Vietnam is over, I'm going to protest by running to the nearest fruit stand and standing there and eating until the war has ended!

I can just hear my friends now. "Look at Brother Greg. He sure is dedicated. He's up to 712 pounds and he's still goin' strong!"

The What of Fasting

What is fasting? It is simply the voluntary withdrawal of food for a period of time. Or, in other words, it is to choose to stop eating.

People go on a mild fast, a very brief fast, every day of their lives and don't even realize it. When you go to bed at night, you don't eat until the next morning. Unless, of course, you get up in the middle of the night and have a midnight snack. But then you don't eat again until you wake up. So there is always a period of say six to eight hours when you don't eat.

When you get up and eat your first meal, what do you call it? Break-fast! When you have your breakfast you are "breaking the fast" of the night before. Your whole body has been resting, including the parts of the body machine which have to work out during the digestive period. Those glands and organs need a period of rest, which means a period when food is not being taken in for them to digest.

The fasting which occurs while you are asleep is only indirectly a voluntary abstaining from food. You don't say, "It's time to stop eating now," but rather, "It's time to go to bed." But it is the result of your body saying to you, "For heaven's sake, go to bed. I need a rest from the further ingestion of food so I can do something with what you've already thrown in here." So your body is making the choice for you.

It is interesting to note that when you go on an extended fast the body requires less and less sleep. The body is not involved in the constant process of exerting energy to digest food, and as more and more waste matter and poisons are eliminated from the system, the body is in need of less rest. The opposite side of that observation is what happens after you eat a big meal, as at Thanksgiving or Christmas. First of all, the meal has probably contained the most impossible combinations of food for your body to handle. You've probably eaten a huge amount of turkey, maybe ham too, untold starches, etc., all of it cooked. So what happens? You go to sleep right after dinner! Your body is so busy trying to handle all that holiday mess you don't even have energy left to walk around.

There is a difference between fasting, starvation and malnutrition. Malnutrition is closer to starvation than to fasting. Malnutrition means "bad nutrition" from the Latin word *malus* meaning "bad, ill." Malnutrition is bad nutrition or "malassimilation," the failure of the body to be able to assimilate and use the food which has been taken in. Malnutrition can be the result of very few scraps of food being eaten, or it can come from large amounts of food being eaten, none of it useful to the body. Well fed but undernourished, in other words. The Ellen H. Richards Institute at Pennsylvania State College concluded in a report that "only one person in a thousand escapes malnutrition."

The marks of malnutrition are the same whether the malnourished person is underfed or overfed. If you look around you, you can see the signs passing by on the street every day. Or perhaps you can use a full-length mirror for the same observation! Two obvious signs of malnutrition are a bloated belly (a "bay window") and a bald head or patches of thin, poor-quality hair. The bloated belly is usually the sign of a diseased colon and the bald or mangy head usually indicates a lack of vitamin B, calcium and protein. Of course, if meat is used as the source of protein, the chances of producing an impacted and diseased colon are greatly increased. In terms of some of the items which will become familiar in the Dick Gregory Natural Diet menu suggestions, protein is supplied by soybeans, pumpkin, squash and sunflower seeds, vitamin B by wheat germ, sunflower seeds, soybeans and sesame seeds, and calcium by kelp, almonds, sesame seeds, soybeans and filberts. As I look over charts of nutritional value of food, I'd say the soybean is the most likely "hair restorer" around.

Starvation occurs when food is denied to the body at a time

when the body is *in need* of sustenance. There is a big difference between the *voluntary withdrawal* from food and the *denial* of food, just as there is a big difference between *true hunger* and plain old hunger, or appetite. When mealtime rolls around we feel "hungry" for all kinds of reasons, not the least of which is that it is part of the eating ritual—mealtime, three times a day. Although we feel "hungry" and have an appetite for food, the body machine is in no way going through the throes of true hunger.

When you get up in the morning, before you break your fast of the night before, if you look in the mirror and stick out your tongue you will notice it is coated. A chalkish coating, sometimes yellowish in color and sometimes white, is on the surface of the tongue. This is an indication that the body is not yet in a state of true hunger, although the chances are you feel "hungry" from force of habit.

If you go on a long fast, the tongue will remain coated during the entire period the body is cleansing itself of impurities. As mentioned in Chapter Two, after the third week of the fast the body will begin a complete overhaul by cleaning out poisons. When that overhaul is completed, the coating on the tongue will disappear, starvation will set in and true hunger will return. Then nourishment must be supplied and denial of food beyond this point would result in death.

After the third or fourth day of a fast, hunger leaves. I don't mean to say you do not get hungry, or experience the nagging pangs of appetite. But *hunger* disappears. It is the mental or ritualistic aspects of eating which are most bothersome. If a person is on a short fast, and one day dinnertime rolls around and that person gives in to the pangs of appetite because he or she has passed a restaurant, or friends are eating, or whatever, invariably the fasting person will say later on in the evening, "Now why did

I do that?" If the person could only have avoided the temptation of the dinner *hour* and its accompanying hunger pangs, the fast could have been continued.

I frequently tell my audiences that sometimes during a fast I have dreams of the "hot dog parade" marching on me! Again, it is appetite playing games with me long before true hunger has set in. It is strange that as certain poisons and stored up wastes begin to be flushed out of the system old tastes return. The "hot dog parade" plagues me though I have long since given up eating hot dogs. Even if I were eating I would parade on past the hot dog stand!

This mental aspect is very important, I believe, in understanding the difference between fasting and starvation. Some people "starve to death" in much shorter periods of time than I, for example, have fasted. I think there are two reasons for this.

First, it is important to drink a lot of water or liquid to assist the process of elimination of waste matter. The person who has been denied food through factors out of his or her control does not look upon the denial of food as a fast. Such a person does not carefully consume the proper amount of water necessary to flush out impurities. And of course such a person does not aid the process of elimination with enemas.

Secondly, the mental attitude is an important factor. When a person chooses to go on a fast, the mind is at ease because the person knows exactly why he or she is refraining from eating. The mental attitude is calm, relaxed and therapeutic. But if a person wants to eat and cannot get any food, the mental attitude is entirely different. Rather than being calm and relaxed, the person is panicked and desperate. The person is worried about starving to death, and I personally believe this mental attitude is a contributing factor when death results. If proper concern is given to the process of elimination and water intake and the mental attitude is calm and relaxed, it is physiologically impossible for a person to die from fasting until Mother Nature gives her clear sign on the tongue.

I would hasten to add one important qualification. If there is an organic disease in the body, to such an extent that the organs involved are damaged beyond the point of their ability to repair themselves during fasting, death may occur during a fast. But fasting is not responsible for the death. Death would have occurred anyway and it just happened to come during the fast. And, as Linda B. Hazzard points out in her book *About Scientific Fasting*, "it is conclusively demonstrated that in a scientifically directed fast, although death in the conditions cited [organs degenerated beyond the stage of repair] cannot be averted, yet because of organic labor lessened, life is prolonged for days or weeks, and distress and pain, if present, are much alleviated."

The Why of Fasting

There are at least three reasons why people may go on a fast— *religious, political* or *scientific* (rational). I do not mean to suggest that the religious and political reasons are irrational, but rather to emphasize that people come to the rational decision that fasting is good and necessary for the body without any political or religious overtones.

Religious fasting is sometimes an act of deprivation of the body as a means of penance for past sins. But when I speak of religious fasting I mean fasting for the purpose of heightened spiritual awareness. It is an act of piety, of freeing oneself from the demands of bodily appetites to be in closer communion with Mother Nature, the Ground of Being, God, the Supreme Being, or whatever name one chooses to call the Universal Force and Intelligence.

Religious fasting is best done in secret—that is, without telling people you are fasting. Jesus called attention to this aspect in the Sermon on the Mount: "Beware of practicing your piety before men in order to be seen by them; for then you will have no reward from your Father who is in heaven." When fasting is done for this purpose, it is best to be in the closest possible contact with Mother Nature. Time should be devoted to being in the open air and sunlight. If possible, one should seek to be near a fresh-water stream or lake or at the seashore and soak and bathe in the tingling freshness of Mother Nature's water. It is also desirable to go into the woods and share communion with Mother Nature's trees and vegetation. The religious fast is an attempt to blend and unite with the created order.

The political fast is public. In my own view, the political fast is more appropriately termed a hunger strike. The political fast is undertaken to call attention to some form of injustice, or to protest a failure to redress just grievances. My own public fasts have been in this hunger-strike category. The political fast is a witness, an example, and a symbol that is shared by all who also protest the particular injustice.

As a witness, it has a public and private effect. When I went on my fast of eating no solid food until the war in Vietnam would be over, I became conscious of the war and its effects more frequently than ever before. For example, any time one of my kids walked through the house eating an apple, my mind immediately focused upon the war in Vietnam. In the same way, people all over the country who knew about my fast, whether they shared my views on the war or not, became conscious of the war when they sat down to a meal.

I personally believe you do not conduct a political fast to make "bad" people "good," or to change the hearts of tyrants and oppressors. Rather, you go on a political fast to provide a rallying point for all of the moral forces and the ethical forces needed to displace the negative forces responsible for the perpetration of a particular injustice.

Scientific or rational fasting is undertaken for the purpose of cleaning out the system, eliminating all toxic poisons collected in the body. It is a detoxification of the body. Scientific fasting is based upon the conviction that toxemia is the basic *cause* of disease. The symptoms of disease that we recognize and seek to treat are really the effects of the body trying to restore itself to a state of health. When we continue to push food into the body as it seeks to heal itself, or shoot chemicals into it, we are forcing the body to use vital energies for purposes other than the restoration of health. Thus, the best way to help the body when the symptoms of disease appear is through fasting, relieving the body of the digestive function, or taking only juices, which provide help in the process of healing.

This all sounds so simple that you cannot help but wonder why fasting is not practiced more universally. Well, a very revealing article from the April 3, 1972, edition of the *Los Angeles Times* by staff writer Murray Seeger indicates that fasting is used in Russia.

The story, datelined Moscow, begins by telling of the experience of Vladimir Leshkovtsev. It seems Vladimir had been treated by doctors for six weeks and told he had infectious metabolic polyarthritis. Poor Vladimir's arthritis got no better, so he decided to take things into his own hands. For forty-five days he ate nothing and drank plentiful supplies of water, and the result was he lost forty-four pounds and his arthritis!

The story goes on to tell of the Moscow Research Institute of

Psychiatry, headed by Dr. Yuri Nikolayev, and its use of "controlled starvation" in treating mental disorders. Other Soviet doctors use "controlled starvation" for treating psoriasis, metabolic disorders, bronchial asthma, hypertension, gallstones, tumors, pancreatitis and early forms of hardening of the arteries.

The Soviet "controlled starvation" treatment is really a twenty-to-forty-day fast. And when we read that it is successfully used in the treatment of "tumors," we get the sneaking suspicion that hidden in the guarded rhetoric of the Soviet story is the assertion that fasting is a possible cure for cancer! Isn't it ironic that we Americans are so concerned about beating the Russians in outer space, while we should be devoting as much time, energy, money and research to finding out about what's happening in our own inner spaces? And it wouldn't take much time or money to discover the miraculous curative powers of fasting.

"Fasting" is a more accurate term than "controlled starvation" because a body system that is in disease not only has no desire for nutriment while in the state of physical imbalance but also has no need for food until it is purified again and able to resume its normal functions.

When we are sick, the desire for food is usually absent. Parents and friends—those most concerned about us—think they are doing us a favor when they urge, "You've got to eat something." And they are fond of reciting the old cliché, "Feed a cold and starve a fever." It is interesting to note how far that particular cliché has strayed from its original wording: "Feed a cold and you'll have to starve a fever!"

One final word about the *Los Angeles Times* story reporting the Soviet experience. Dr. Nikolayev was asked, "Why is self-imposed starvation healthful when involuntary starvation is harmful?" The difference, the good doctor replied, is that under involuntary starvation the body dies from poisons contained within itself!

"In our cases," Dr. Nikolayev continued, "we try by all means to withdraw endotoxins from the body as soon as possible. Altogether, we have treated some 7,000 patients at our clinic. Our extensive experience enables us to broaden the range of application of this method and to take up the treatment of cases formerly considered hopeless."

End of quote!

The Who of Fasting

To trace the history of fasting would take an entire volume, more likely a series. But I suppose the history of fasting begins with the instinctive tendency of animals to fast when sick. In both the Old and New Testaments of the Bible, fasting is a frequently mentioned activity. Moses fasted forty days, as did Jesus. The Hebrew prophets and the apostles engaged in prayer and fasting. The Pharisees, a Hebrew sect at the time of Jesus, practiced semiweekly fasts.

The Roman theologian Tertullian wrote a treatise on fasting in A.D. 210. Earlier, in A.D. 110, Polycarp urged fasting as a means of warding off temptation and lust. The Druid priests among the Celts were required to undergo a probationary period of prolonged fasting before initiation into the mysteries of their cult. In the Mithraic or sun-worshiping religion of Persia a fifty-day fast was required.

It is reported that Egyptian hospitals at the time of the French occupation by Napoleon were using fasting as a treatment for venereal disease. Avicenna, the Arabian physician of the tenth and eleventh centuries, prescribed three-week fasts for his patients, especially as a cure for smallpox and syphilis.

In the mid-nineteenth century, therapeutic fasting began to come to the attention of many through the treatment of Dr. Isaac Jennings of Oberlin, Ohio. Others continued to spread the word of the benefits of fasting, including Sylvester Graham, Dr. Edward Hooker, Dr. Henry Tanner and Bernarr Macfadden. Dr. Tanner, for example, undertook an experimental fast in Chicago in the mid-nineteenth century at the age of fifty. He fasted forty-three days. Ten years later he fasted fifty days. The thin gray hair he had when he began the first fast had been replaced by a thick crop of black hair by the time of his second fast. He died at the ripe old age of ninety-three.

Gandhi is probably the most famous practitioner of the political fast. But more recently many others have fasted for varying lengths of time for political purposes, including the Reverend Charles Koen of Cairo, Illinois, Robert Williams, H. Rap Brown, Cesar Chavez, David Dellinger, Paul Mayer and, at the time this book is going into production, Sean MacStiofain.

The When of Fasting

In discussing the "when" of fasting, we must make a distinction between the long fast and the short-term fast—what we might call an "extended breakfast." It is very good for cleaning out the body to go on a twenty-four-hour or a thirty-six-hour fast once every week. This can be from dinner to dinner, lunch to lunch, or whatever you choose during the twenty-four-hour fast. The thirty-six-hour fast would be from lunch to dinner the following day, or dinner to breakfast thirty-six hours later. During this period of time, only fresh, pure water is taken, in very plentiful supplies. This means no fruit or vegetable juices. You may add a teaspoon of freshly squeezed lemon juice to each glass of water and sweeten with honey. Persons suffering from diabetes should use tupelo honey, which is available at the health food store. The first meal after breaking the twenty-four- or thirty-six-hour fast should be a raw vegetable salad, like grated carrots and cabbage, which will act as a broom sweeping out the intestines and colon.

Dr. Otto H. F. Buchinger in his book *About Fasting* offers an extended list of ailments which make it advisable for a sufferer to go on a longer fast, two weeks or more. Some of them are as follows:

1. Metabolism disorders like overweight and underweight, rheumatism, the initial stages of diabetes.
2. Diseases of the heart, circulation and blood vessels such as high and low blood pressure, coronary thrombosis, early cases of arteriosclerosis.
3. Skin diseases like psoriasis, eczema, acne, boils.
4. Diseases of the digestive organs like loss of appetite, liver and gall bladder difficulties, diarrhea, stubborn constipation.
5. Diseases of the respiratory organs, chills, asthma, aftereffects of pneumonia attacks.
6. Kidney and bladder disorders.
7. Female complaints like menopausal symptoms, disturbances in the menstrual flow, chronic inflammations of the womb.
8. Allergies and nervous complaints like nervous exhaustion, migraine, recurring headache, neuritis, neuralgia, insomnia, depression, sexual weakness or overstimulation.

The above list is by no means complete, but it is an indication of the great variety of illnesses which might be relieved by a prolonged cleansing fast.

Thus, the when of fasting depends upon the individual. When

your mind and body are convinced that you have been disobeying Mother Nature, an extended fast may be in order.

The How of Fasting

Once the decision to put the body on an extended fast has been made, certain preparatory steps should be taken. The most important is to start the cleansing process in the body which will be intensified during the fast. It is advisable to go on a diet of only fruit juice for at least a week before starting the complete fast. If the decision is made well enough in advance, you could begin by eating only fruit for a week, then going to fruit juice and finally into the fast. During this preparatory period for the fast, it would be a good idea to start taking enemas, every other day or every third day.

When the fast has begun, only pure water will be taken. The best water is rain water that has been warmed by the direct light and rays of the sun. Distilled water may also be used, but never use fluoridated tap water.

The water consumed should not be too hot or too cold. Room temperature is all right, though some fasting authorities insist upon body temperature (98.6 degrees Fahrenheit). Water should be taken when thirsty or hungry. Every attempt should be made to take as much water as possible; a gallon a day is good. Do not give up the water consumption even if you are "turned off" by water at some point during the fast.

Once the fast has begun, daily enemas should be taken to assist the process of flushing out impurities in the body. Remember you may add the strained juice of two or three lemons, a little honey and/or blackstrap molasses if available.

Daily bathing is also important during the fast. Take tub baths in preference to showers if at all possible. The body is flushing impurities out through the pores of the skin so bathing is very important. A bath in the morning and a bath in the evening before retiring are sufficient. I would not take more than three baths daily. Never use a harsh soap when bathing. The morning bath might be with Epsom salts rather than soap (use two pounds of Epsom salts for a tub of water), and the evening bath with a natural soap from the health food store (coconut, cucumber, etc.) or Ivory soap. Massage the body gently when bathing.

It is also very important to keep the body warm during the long fast. If you go to work, remember to dress warmly, especially in the summer if you work around air-conditioning. At home you should avoid air-conditioning and never sleep in an air-conditioned room.

Light exercise, such as moderate walking, is all right during the fasting period. Do not lift anything during a long fast, and avoid sudden movements, like getting up suddenly or changing positions suddenly. Sometimes people make such sudden movements, experience a feeling of dizziness and take it as a sign to break the fast. Remember the cleansing process the body is going through, especially the cleansing of the bloodstream, and you will realize the sudden movement was merely a shock to the system in the process of renewing itself.

I hate to mention it but it *is* important to practice celibacy (no sex) during a water fast, a week before and two weeks after. But don't be too depressed. You'll be a lot better at it once the body is purified! Nothing can beat pure sex.

When breaking the fast, only fruit juice should be consumed, one day of it for every five days you were fasting. Thus, in breaking a forty-day fast, fruit juice should be taken for eight days. The fruit juice should be heated like soup. Grape juice from the bottle may be used. It sounds like a contradiction, I know, since the pasteurizing process will have destroyed the enzymes. But during the fasting period, those little villi will have actually fallen asleep. The fresh enzymes in the pure fruit juice would be too much of a shock for the sleeping villi—like throwing ice-cold water in a sleeping person's face!

It is very, very important to break your fast correctly. While it is not possible to die on the fast (except under the special conditions mentioned earlier), it is possible to do extreme or even mortal damage by breaking the fast incorrectly.

Of course, it should go without saying that the kind of diet you adopt permanently after the long fast will determine the real benefits of fasting. After the long fast and the cleansing it brings, you should go on a natural diet of raw foods and increasingly more fruit. It's the only way to stay clean, look young, feel even younger and be around for the twenty-first-century action!

The Result of Fasting

The long fast puts the *entire* body through a cleansing. That also includes toxic accumulations in the brain. And as the brain is cleansed the mind is released. During a long fast you will notice a heightening of ethical and spiritual awareness.

One of the things that happen during a long, cleansing fast is that you lose the six basic fears which plague humankind:

Fear of poverty
Fear of death
Fear of sickness
Fear of getting old
Fear of being criticized
Fear of losing your love

All six, or some combination of these fears, haunt everyone who is captive to the usual nervous imbalances accompanying toxic diet. But when those fears disappear you are really at home with Mother Nature and happily at peace with life in Mother Nature's world. You can shout the words of the familiar freedom phrase and they will have a meaning only you will truly realize: "Free at last!"

8

Mother Nature's Medicare

Chapter Five was primarily a "shopping list." This chapter might be viewed as a "prescription," emphasizing as it does the fantastic benefits and curative powers available to anyone who conscientiously listens to Mother Nature. Most people don't realize that relief from "disease" is easily available. For the price of a juicer and raw vegetables and fruits, folks can treat themselves for most ailments.

Instead, you go to a doctor, who gives you a prescription you can't even read. So you take it to some druggist and get it read for you. You've got to trust him (or her)! For all you know, the doctor and the druggist might have a thing going for them. The note might say, "Hey, baby. There's nothing wrong with this cat at all. Just lay some candy on him and charge him thirty dollars. I'll be by after the office closes for my cut."

Doctors can play games with us naïve human beings. We go into a doctor's office and the first thing the doctor says is, "What's wrong with you?" If you knew that you wouldn't be there!

That's why I'd feel better going to a veterinarian. The vet has to know what he's doing because animals can't talk. If a big old elephant puts his foot on the vet's chest, the vet better not make a mistake. If a veterinarian asked a gorilla to point to where it hurts, he might just demonstrate!

Getting Juiced

Mother Nature provides a complete "pharmacy" of health-restoring medicines, available without prescription. There is a simple rule for understanding raw juices. Fruit juices are the cleansers and vegetable juices are the builders. Fruit juices break down mucus and clean out the system, and vegetable juices build cells and tissues. Vegetable juices can also be helpful in cleaning out the body, however, by building up glands and organs and enabling them to perform their natural functions.

Isn't it odd that some folks refer to drinking too much alcohol as "getting juiced"? Of course, if they *really* got juiced more often, with raw fruit and vegetable juices, they'd soon lose their taste for alcohol. Let me suggest some concoctions, and remember, fruit and vegetable *juices* can be mixed and taken together. It is not the same as eating raw fruits and vegetables at the same time, a practice I've warned against.

PARTY TIME

Having a party? Try serving a drink made of ½ pint orange juice, 3 tablespoons strawberry juice, 1 tablespoon lemon juice, 2 tablespoons honey and ½ pint water. Mix well. That makes a quart, which should serve about eight folks. So readjust your mixtures according to the number of guests.

Or try this party pleaser. Mix equal parts carrot, celery and apple juice and a teaspoon of honey (for a quart).

Planning a wedding reception? Instead of champagne, use nature's champagne: mix 3 parts pineapple juice and 1 part cucumber juice and a teaspoon of orange juice (for a quart). Or add orange juice to taste.

HEADACHE

Got a headache? Instead of an aspirin, mix 2 parts tomato juice to 1 part celery juice and add 2 teaspoons onion juice. Take every couple of hours until the headache disappears.

UPSET STOMACH?

Did you "make a big mistake"? Instead of dropping two tablets into a glass of water and watching them fizz, mix equal amounts of celery and orange juice and a teaspoon of lemon juice. Sweeten with honey if you want to. Or you can take fresh spinach juice alone. Or 5 parts carrot juice to 3 parts spinach juice. Or 10 parts carrot juice to 3 parts each of beet and cucumber juices.

NERVOUS?

Don't take a tranquilizer! Mix ½ cup each of celery, parsley, turnip leaf and carrot juices. Add a teaspoon of fresh lemon juice.

SENIOR CITIZEN SIP

To stay younger longer, combine 2 parts carrot juice with 1 part each of cucumber and cabbage juices. Add orange and lemon juices to taste. Drink a glassful morning and evening.

NIGHTCAP

For those who suffer from insomnia, can't sleep, get up tired, and stay that way all day, celery juice is the answer. Or it can be taken in combination with carrot juice—5 parts carrot to 3 parts celery.

ONCE-A-DAY MULTIPLE VITAMIN LIQUID

Instead of capsules or tablets, drink at least a pint a day of a mixture of 4 ounces carrot juice, 2 ounces celery juice and 2 ounces apple juice. It's much tastier than a tablet!

Wonder Slugs

Whenever I'm reading or writing anything that lists diseases, I'm reminded of my army days. It is very depressing when you take the physical examination for military service. You are given a form to fill out which is forty pages of nothing but diseases! Then at the end of the list it says, "Others."

I thought I had a way to beat the service. I went down the whole list of diseases and checked "yes" beside every one of them. Then on the last category—"Others"—I wrote "Whooping polio—twice." The recruiting sergeant took my form, looked it over and said, "You're just the type of soldier we're looking for—the kind that can't be killed."

Instead of filling up with the latest so-called miracle drugs, try several "wonder slugs" of fresh raw juice. Drinking at least a pint a day will help the body in its constant struggle to return to a normal condition. But in cases of serious troubles, the more raw juice the better, a quart or more a day.

There are many arguments in favor of getting into the raw juice habit. One's the "toothless" argument. Folks with dentures, bad teeth or no teeth at all can handle juices quite easily. Then there's the "executive" argument. Folks with ulcers or no time to sit down and chew a meal properly can get a large, nourishing salad meal in juice form. Or there's the "sickroom" argument. Folks who have lost their appetite, especially invalids, can get all their nourishment in liquid form when they can't face the prospect of stuffing down solid food. And finally there's the "pint or peck" argument. You can get so much more nourishment and consume so many more vegetables or fruits in juice form. It would be a real chore to consume a half peck of raw fruits or vegetables. Yet some doctors prescribe a gallon of raw juice a day to their patients in serious cases. The juice retains all of the vitamins and minerals of the fruit or vegetable, so that large quantities of juice revitalize an ailing system in an amazingly short period of time.

Let me hasten to add that my suggested juice remedies are not formal prescriptions. First of all, they are not written in Latin. Also, the law requires that a person must be licensed to offer medical prescriptions. Neither of my two doctorates is in the area of medicine. What is said here about Mother Nature's "wonder slugs" is simply for information. Do with it what you will, though I would remind you it has been the experience of many people to return to complete health by using raw juice therapy.

Beet juice is one of the more underrated items in Mother Nature's pharmacy. How many times have you heard someone describe an embarrassing situation with the phrase, "I turned red as a beet!" White readers will have heard it more than I have. Folks have two favorite ways of describing something reddish in color—"blood red" and "beet red."

There is a close relationship between blood and beets, as beet juice is one of the best resources for building up the red blood corpuscles and toning up the body generally. The use of beet juice in treating cases of anemia, low blood pressure, poor circulation, low vitality and suppressed menstruation has been very successful.

It is also a good blood cleanser and is often used to treat eczema and psoriasis.

Surprisingly, the actual iron content of the beet is not high. And we all know from television commercials that if you've got "tired blood" you need more iron. Right? Wrong! Not in the case of beets. The sodium content in the beet is more than 50 percent, while the calcium content is about 5 percent. This proportion is valuable in maintaining the solubility of calcium. When eating cooked foods has caused considerable inorganic calcium to form deposits in the blood vessels, causing such ailments as varicose veins and hardening of the arteries, the liberal use of beet juice will help to dissolve them. The chlorine content of beet juice serves as a cleanser of the liver, the kidneys and the gall bladder, as well as stimulating lymph activity throughout the body.

Beet juice is also good for the heart and it has apparently been successfully used to treat tumors. John B. Lust, in his book *About Raw Juices,* tells of the work of Dr. S. Firenczi, director of a country clinic in Csorna, Hungary. Dr. Firenczi began giving his tumor patients red beets as a treatment in October 1960. (The treatment had been used in 1938 for leukemia cases by a man named Kunstmann.) Dr. Firenczi found that fifteen out of sixteen cases were successfully arrested, with weight gained, blood count changing for the better and cancerous growths reduced.

When juicing beets, it is good to include some of the beet tops. But it is best not to drink more than a wineglassful at a time, since greater quantities sometimes produce nausea or dizziness, possibly caused by the rapid cleansing effect upon the liver.

Carrot juice, or carrots themselves, are usually associated with improving eyesight. As the old line says, "You never saw a rabbit wearing glasses, did you?" But there's more to carrot juice than meets the eyes! It is one of the richest available sources of vitamin A. And it also contains ample quantities of vitamins B, C, D, E, G and K, as well as the minerals calcium, copper, magnesium, potassium, sodium, phosphorus, chlorine, sulfur and iron.

Vitamin A is especially important for keeping the mucous membranes in a healthy condition. The mucous membranes line all the cavities of the body. They consist of two layers, the top one composed of billions of cells and the lower having extremely pliable and elastic muscle fibers. A vitamin A deficiency obstructs the normal secretion of disinfectant mucus, affecting the bladder, the kidneys, the alimentary tract, the mouth, tonsils, sinuses, tongue, eyes, ear canal or tear ducts.

Carrot juice is also a great aid to the liver. Sometimes after drinking large quantities of carrot juice, folks observe a discoloration of the skin. They become alarmed and think the carrot juice is causing jaundice or something. It is really a sign that the liver is cleaning itself out. The material clogging the liver is passed into the lymph for elimination through the pores of the skin. The waste material has a distinctly orange or yellowish color. So the discoloration of the skin is a welcome sign that the liver is returning to health.

Vitamin A deficiency manifests itself in some of these symptoms: dry, scaly or rough skin (especially on the arms and legs); diarrhea or other intestinal disorders; no appetite; growth retardation; weight loss; lack of vigor or downright weakness; poor teeth; stones in the kidney and bladder; and it may be a factor in sterility!

An eight-ounce glass of carrot juice will provide about 50,000 units or more of vitamin A. The liver has the capacity to store up large amounts of vitamin A and draw upon the storehouse when it is needed.

Vitamin E is also available in large amounts from carrot juice.

In experiments with sterile animals, vitamin E helped them over-come their sterility and reproduce once again. A word to the wise should be sufficient. Drink carrot juice and you *shall* overcome!

Always wash carrots thoroughly before juicing them, using a stiff vegetable brush. You may scrape them lightly, but don't peel! Valuable vitamins and minerals are lying close to the surface. The juice should be consumed immediately after it is made. If not, keep the juice under refrigeration in tightly screwed jars to pre-vent oxidation.

Cucumber juice is much better than beer in promoting the flow of urine. It is the best natural diuretic known. It is a natural hair restorer, particularly when mixed with carrot, lettuce and spinach juices (7 ounces carrot to 2 ounces each of lettuce, spinach and cucumber), because of its high silicon and sulfur content. Cucum-ber juice contains more than 40 percent potassium, 10 percent sodium, 7 percent calcium, 20 percent phosphorus and 7 percent chlorine. It is also excellent for the skin and nails.

Thus, the CBC cocktail (carrot, beet and cucumber juices), one of the remedies listed earlier for an upset stomach, is a potent an-tidote for many ailments which eventually end up being treated with the surgical knife, such as gall and kidney stones, appendici-tis, tumors and tonsillitis. It is also helpful in treating such varied disturbances as bed-wetting, measles, gout and gonorrhea!

Cabbage juice is a particularly effective treatment for ulcer trou-bles. Dr. Alvenia Fulton is a living testimony to the healing power of cabbage juice. In 1955 she was hospitalized with bleeding duo-denal ulcers. Surgery was urged by her doctors but she refused to permit it. For thirteen days Dr. Fulton consumed a quart of fresh cabbage juice each day—and she was cured! She continued a diet of raw salads and fruits and her ulcers never returned.

Cabbage juice is high in both sulfur and chlorine content, as well as being a relatively good source of iodine. When combined with raw carrot juice, it forms an excellent source of vitamin C, an important factor in maintaining healthy gums. Cabbage juice alone contains a vitamin composition which is particularly healthy for the mucous membrane of the intestinal tract and stomach. However, this vitamin component is quickly destroyed by heat. One hundred and twenty pounds of cooked or canned cabbage could not furnish the same vital food value as one-half pint of straight raw cabbage juice. So the Fighting Irish can't get their strength from the traditional Saint Patrick's Day corned beef and cabbage dinner!

If an apple a day keeps the doctor away, *apple juice* in the morn makes the doctor forlorn! Unless, of course, the doctor is more interested in the health of individuals than in customers. Apple juice contains nine out of the sixteen chemical elements required by the human body and four of the six most important ones. It is easily assimilated by the body and, taken each morning, helps to encourage elimination and tone up the system. It is rich in vitamin C and, working harmoniously with vitamin A, also found in apple juice, it wards off infections in the stomach and intestines.

Apple juice should be made fresh daily. Before running the cut apples through the juice extractor, pour a little lemon or pineapple juice over them to prevent them from turning brown. When juicing apples, the core and skin should be put through the juicing machine, as they contain valuable minerals. Two to eight pints of apple juice may be taken daily; and when taken at night, apple juice soothes the nerves and helps to promote sound sleep.

Apple juice combines well with other juices. Half apple and half carrot juice is an excellent tonic from Mother Nature's pharmacy. Or 5 ounces apple juice combined with 6 ounces carrot juice and 5 ounces celery juice will give the body necessary sodium (salt) content. Celery juice is rich in sodium and is an especially good hot weather drink used in place of salt tablets. Heavy smokers should also use celery juice to help rid themselves of carbon dioxide. More important, of course, they should quit smoking. And apple juice also combines well with spinach juice—6 ounces apple to 8 ounces carrot and 2 ounces spinach. This combination is very good for anyone suffering from bleeding gums.

Apple cider vinegar also is therapeutic. While the distilled or wine vinegar found on the supermarket shelf contains acetic acid, which is very harmful to the red blood corpuscles, causing anemia in some cases when the amount of acid is high, pure apple cider vinegar contains malic acid, a constructive acid which combines with alkaline elements in the body to produce energy or to be stored up for future use as glycogen. Apple cider vinegar has an external medicinal effect as well. It can be used as an antiseptic. In Scotland, it used to be common practice to apply apple cider vinegar to varicose veins, morning and night. The patient also drank two or three glasses of water with two teaspoons of apple cider vinegar. The veins shrank!

There are many, many other raw juice remedies in Mother Nature's pharmacy. I urge you to try to get one of the books on the subject listed in the bibliography at the end of this book. The old home remedies your grandparents used to practice frequently were based on the soundness of Mother Nature's principles. You'll find that the old folks were hip!

Let me close with a reminder to any skeptics who might be tempted to scoff at the idea of raw juice therapy and prefer still to patronize the corner drugstore. It is not at all unusual for scoffing and ridicule to greet unfamiliar ideas. Copernicus was almost burned at the stake because he dared to make the silly claim that the earth revolved around the sun. Folks thought Columbus was crazy because he said the world wasn't flat. Giordano Bruno *was* executed for running around telling folks that other suns existed. Isaac Newton held back publishing his theories for fear of being laughed at by his colleagues. William Harvey felt the same way and waited twelve years before getting up enough nerve to say he thought the heart pumps blood through the circulatory system. Folks called him a crackpot and laughed him out of the medical business.

It's never easy for folks to accept the simple, natural truths, especially when they are *so* simple and *so* natural that people are ashamed of not knowing them. But just remember, Mother Nature was using hearts to pump blood for a mighty long time before William Harvey even thought about it. Her healing principles have never changed. And when you really think about it, I'll bet in *your* heart you know she's right!

9

Dick Gregory's
Weight On/Weight Off
Natural Diet

One of the founding fathers of these United States, old Brother Benjamin Franklin, came up with a right-on line when he observed, "A full belly is the mother of all evil." And another great American, Tom Edison, made the electrifying suggestion, "People gorge themselves with rich foods, use their time, ruin their digestion, and poison themselves. . . ."

So in the spirit of '76 and the electric light bulb, let me offer the Dick Gregory Weight On/Weight Off Natural Diet. The menu suggestions which follow incorporate my understanding of proper food combinations and nutritional needs. In this chapter I've included a diet for folks who want to lose weight, one for those who want to gain weight, and one for those who aren't particularly concerned about weight at all but just want to get things right between themselves and Mother Nature. If you don't fit any of those categories, try the chapter on pets!

Equipment

You'll need some basic equipment to follow and prepare the Natural Diet. We'll start with the cheaper items and work up to those more expensive.

Orange Juice Squeezer: You can get an orange juice squeezer for about any price you want to pay. At the supermarket you'll find all kinds of very inexpensive hand squeezers. And if you want to invest more you can get a mechanized squeezer which requires less elbow grease. You'll need your squeezer for preparing orange, grapefruit, tangerine, lemon and lime juices.

Strainer: This is another inexpensive item. You'll need it for straining out the pulp and seeds from juices when advisable.

Grinder and Grater: There are many varieties of grinders and graters. You'll need a grinder for grinding nuts, for example. At the supermarket you can get either a hand grinder-grater or a nut mill for a little over a dollar.

Chopper and Shredder: You'll find a chopper and a shredder helpful in the preparation of salads. These are also relatively inexpensive supermarket items. Or you can get a Kitchen Magician at the five-and-dime store for about ten bucks.

Blender: Now we begin to move into the more expensive items. A blender is very, very important to the convenient and proper preparation of the Natural Diet. Blenders vary greatly in price, depending upon the number of speeds and so on. However, I do know from conversations with company executives that Sears, Roebuck and Company now offers a blender for about twelve dollars.

Juicer: Juicers also vary tremendously in price. Sears has two relatively low-priced manually operated models available either at the local store or from the catalogue department. One is the Helical Grinder, which sells for about eighteen dollars. It is a meat and food chopper, but it has an attachment for juice extracting. The other is the Squeezo Press, a hand press selling for about twenty-five dollars, and it is used in making sauces and purées. It is not basically a juice extractor.

More expensive electric juicers are the Champion, manufactured by Plastaket Manufacturing Company, Lodi, California, 95240, and the AEG Juice Extractor, available from the Phoenix Juicer Company, 30 Vesey Street, New York, New York, 10007. Two other juicers in the high-priced category are the Acme and the Atlas.

The advantage of the more expensive juicers is their ability to liberate the hidden values from the fibers of fruits and vegetables; in other words to track the life line and provide the full nutritional value of the fruit or vegetable in liquid form.

Other manually operated inexpensive juicers are also manufactured, though they are probably more available in small towns and rural areas. If price is a bothersome factor, it is worth looking around.

If all else fails, you can do wonders with a piece of muslin cloth. Fruits such as grape, orange, lemon, grapefruit and tomato have an abundance of juice. Cut the fruits into small pieces and then squeeze the little pieces tightly in the muslin cloth, letting the juice drop in a glass or bowl. The citrus fruits should first be peeled. Carrot juice may be made by first grating the carrots finely into a soft mush, then squeezing the mush through the muslin cloth.

So much for equipment. But before going any further, I want to offer a political suggestion. Perhaps a senator or congressman/woman will read these pages and follow up on it. I see no reason at all why a juicer and a blender should not be tax-deductible items.

Medical expenses are tax deductible. If pills, chemicals and medicines are allowed to be written off income tax, certainly a juicer
and a blender should also be allowed to be a write-off. A juicer
and a blender are both legitimate *medical expenses* as they are used
to prepare the very best medicine of all, Mother Nature's raw fruit
and vegetable health restorers.

Optimum Diet

The Dick Gregory Diet is not a calorie counter's diet. Nor does
it claim to be a "balanced" diet. The term "balanced diet" is both
overworked and misused. It really is meaningless. Think of the
"balanced diet charts" you see hanging in the hygiene classrooms
in schools—pictures of cows and pigs and slabs of bacon, eggs,
cheese, milk, etc. The vegetables, fruits and juices are there also,
but you have to get past the steaks and chops to see them.

Rather than the term "balanced diet," I would suggest *optimum diet.* That is, the menus in this chapter and those that
follow are designed to give optimum nutritional value rather
than a balanced variety among all the potential things that can
be eaten in this world! And optimum nutritional value is the
primary consideration for overweight folks, underweight folks,
folks with special health problems, athletes, healthy kids and
everyone who eats.

Though it may seem strange to couple "weight on" and "weight
off" in the same chapter heading, the overweight person and the
underweight person are both suffering from *malnutrition.* They
are undernourished. Well fed, or frequently fed, perhaps. But undernourished just the same. They are not getting the optimum
nutritional value from the foods they are taking in. The big bay
window, or bloated stomach, is more of a sign of malnutrition

than a skinny emaciated form. Both the overweight and the underweight person need a good cleansing of the system so that their intake of proper foods can be assimilated and used by the body.

Persons trying to gain weight so often try to do it by eating foods that "will make them fat." They eat ice cream, cake, pie, pastries, potatoes, starches by the carload, and so on. The truth of the matter is, as the Body Owner's Manual made quite clear, they are starving their bodies and vital organs by stuffing in foods that cannot possibly be used, lining the intestines with mucus, for example, and preventing the absorption of digested foods. And they wonder why they can't put on weight. Their bodies wonder why they can't quit.

You can't put on weight by eating food the body cannot use. It is not the *quantity* of food but rather the *quality* of food which allows the body to build itself up to the desired weight. Paavo Airola, in his book *There Is a Cure for Arthritis*, writes:

The latest scientific research shows that the single most important health and longevity factor is a scanty diet or underfeeding. Statistics collected from the several thousands of centenarians in Russia show that one common characteristic of all people who lived 100 years or longer is that throughout their lives they were all moderate eaters. Extensive animal studies reveal that moderate underfeeding increases longevity and decreases incidence of degenerative diseases. The eminent scientist, Dr. C. M. McCay of Cornell University, has shown by his research that overeating is the major cause of premature aging in civilized countries. To prolong life and assure good health he recommends a scanty diet of nutritionally superior natural foods.

If you still want to put on some weight, I am about to tell you the optimum nutritional way to do it. But first let me present recipes for salad dressings and soy, seed and nut milk which are to be used in all of the natural diets.

Salad Dressing Recipes

LEMONAISE

Mix and beat together 2 teaspoons almonds or pecans, flaked very fine, with 1 tablespoon lemon juice. Let mixture stand 15 minutes or more. Then add 2 tablespoons olive oil and beat well into a cream. The flavor of the cream may be enhanced to taste by adding ½ teaspoon of caraway seeds, aniseed or mustard seed. Use your blender for mixing if you have one.

FRUIT DRESSING

Mix well 3 tablespoons lemon juice, 3 tablespoons orange juice, 1 tablespoon honey and 4 tablespoons olive oil, pour into a jar and shake well.

AVOCADO DRESSING

Mash the pulp of one avocado. Add the juice of 1 orange or 1 lemon very gradually to season. Whip with a rotary beater until the consistency of whipped cream. Add a little honey to the mixture if used on a fruit salad, or some finely grated onion if used on a vegetable salad.

FRENCH DRESSING

Combine ½ cup olive oil, ¼ cup lemon juice, the juice of 1 tomato or ¼ cup tomato juice (freshly squeezed). Mix all ingredients thoroughly (use blender if available).

OIL AND APPLE JUICE

Add ½ cup fresh apple juice to 2 ounces olive oil. Shake or beat together.

OIL AND LEMON JUICE

Shake or beat together ½ cup lemon juice, 2 ounces olive oil and
1 teaspoon honey. Orange juice may be substituted for the lemon
juice for a variation.

TOMATO NUT

Mix together ½ cup tomatoes, peeled and mashed, ¼ cup almonds
or pecans, finely flaked. Use blender if available. A little olive oil may
also be added.

HERB DRESSING

Combine 1 cup soy or olive oil; ⅓ cup lemon juice; ¼ teaspoon each
oregano, basil, thyme, garlic and paprika. Mix well in the blender with
two tablespoons honey.

Health Milk Recipes

SOYBEAN MILK

Use ½ to 1 cup of soybeans per quart of water. Wash beans thoroughly
and soak overnight. Keep the water and liquefy in a blender. To strain,
squeeze thoroughly through a muslin cloth or a cheesecloth. Sweeten
with honey. This recipe for soy milk is excellent for baby formulas.

SESAME SEED MILK

Combine ½ cup sesame seeds, 1 tablespoon honey, 1½ cups pure
water. Mix in the blender at high speed for about five minutes. Strain
through a cheesecloth or muslin cloth into a large bowl. Sesame milk
should be made fresh daily.

NUT MILK

Combine 1 cup almonds or pecans, 2 cups pure water, 1 tablespoon honey. If desired, the almonds may be soaked for a period of time and the outer covering scraped or washed off. Blend ingredients at high speed for about five minutes. Nut milk should be made fresh daily and served immediately. It should not stand more than three or four hours.

Dick Gregory's Weight-On Diet

You will notice that some of the menus suggested call for steamed vegetables. I can hear you saying now, "I thought you didn't believe in cooking food." I don't! But steaming vegetables is not the same as boiling the life and nutrition out of them. When steaming vegetables, it is best to use as little water as possible, letting them steam in their own juices. A steaming basket or double-boiler are helpful items to have. If the vegetables are cooked directly over the fire, keep the fire very low. Vegetables should be stirred constantly until their juices change to steam and then covered tight and let steam a short time.

MENU I

Breakfast

- Tall glass of freshly squeezed grapefruit juice.
- Soak old-fashioned rolled oats and dried prunes, figs and/or apricots in pure water overnight.
  Before serving, add a tablespoon of wheat germ and sweeten with honey.
- Glass of soy milk, seed milk or nut milk.

Lunch

- Large salad of mixed vegetables—lettuce, celery, carrots, radishes—topped with kelp, caraway seed, sunflower seed or sesame seed.
- Lemonaise or one of the other dressings may be used as a topping.

Dinner

- Tall glass of fresh carrot or other vegetable juice.
- Steamed turnip greens or spinach, squash or beets.
  Sprinkle sesame seed or sunflower seed for topping.
- Almonds or raisins may be used for dessert.
- Cup of alfalfa or mint tea.

MENU II
....

Breakfast

- Tall glass of freshly squeezed grapefruit juice.
- Dish of berries in season, or fresh fruit sprinkled with a tablespoon or two of wheat germ.
- Cup of rosemary, peppermint or anise tea.

Lunch

- Tall glass of fresh orange, tomato or other fruit juice.
- Soaked dried figs, prunes and raisins mixed with ½ cup ground almonds and a tablespoon of wheat germ.
- Glass of soy, seed or nut milk.

Dinner

- Tall glass of fresh carrot or other vegetable juice.
- Steamed string beans with flaked almonds.
- Steamed shredded beets and carrots.
- Cup of alfalfa or mint tea.

MENU III

Breakfast

- Tall glass of fresh orange juice.
- Old-fashioned rolled oats soaked overnight.
- Dried prunes, figs and/or apricots soaked overnight.
- Add 1 or 2 tablespoons of wheat germ and sweeten with honey before serving.
- Glass of soy, seed or nut milk.

Lunch

- Tall glass of freshly squeezed grapefruit juice.
- Large mixed vegetable salad—lettuce, carrots, celery—topped with sesame seed, sunflower seed or pumpkin seed, with lemonaise or other salad dressing.
- Glass of soy, seed or nut milk.

Dinner

- Tall glass of fresh carrot or other vegetable juice.
- Cabbage salad: Shred equal parts red, white and green cabbage and combine with finely chopped carrot.
  Add a teaspoon of dill seed and mix together.
  Top with pumpkin or sunflower seed and use lemonaise or one of the other dressings to moisten.
- Cup of alfalfa or mint tea.

MENU IV

Breakfast

- Tall glass of freshly squeezed grapefruit juice.
- Sliced fresh peaches or pears.

- 4 ounces yogurt mixed with ¼ cup sunflower seeds and ¼ cup finely ground pumpkin seeds and 1 tablespoon honey.
- Cup of mint tea.

Lunch
- Tall glass of fresh carrot or other fresh vegetable juice.
- A large tomato stuffed with yogurt and chopped nuts, like almonds, or seeds.
  Sprinkle with wheat germ.
- An apple may be eaten for dessert.
- Glass of soy, seed or nut milk.

Dinner
- Tall glass of fresh vegetable juice.
- Steamed cabbage topped with caraway seeds and/or sunflower or sesame seeds.
- Steamed beets and steamed cauliflower may be served in combination.
- Cup of alfalfa or mint tea.

MENU V

Breakfast
- Tall glass of freshly squeezed orange or grapefruit juice.
- Sliced bananas sprinkled with wheat germ.
  Add tablespoon of honey and top with sprinkled almonds.
- Glass of soy, seed or nut milk.

Lunch
- Tall glass of fresh carrot or other freshly made vegetable juice.
- Shredded cabbage and grated carrot salad.

Mix in minced onion and minced parsley.

Top with lemonaise or one of the other dressings and serve on romaine lettuce.

Pumpkin, sesame and sunflower seeds may also be added to taste.

- Glass of soy, seed or nut milk.

Dinner

- Glass of fresh vegetable juice.
- Steamed asparagus, steamed beets, steamed okra.

  You may want to grate the beets.

  Top with sunflower seeds or sesame seeds.
- Cup of mint tea.
- Later in the evening, have some raisins and an apple.

MENU VI

Breakfast

- Tall glass of freshly squeezed orange or grapefruit juice.
- Dish of peaches, berries in season or melon with 2 tablespoons wheat germ, 2 tablespoons ground almonds, 1 tablespoon honey.
- Glass of soy, seed or nut milk.

Lunch

- Tall glass of fresh carrot juice (or other fresh vegetable juice).
- 2 cups cubed apples, 1 cup raisins and 1 cup chopped almonds mixed together with the juice of a lemon.

  Add honey if desired.
- Glass of soy, seed or nut milk, or cup of herb tea.

Dinner

- Tall glass of fresh vegetable juice.

- Mixed vegetable salad—lettuce, celery, parsley (chopped) and radishes—mixed with sesame seeds and topped with herb dressing.
- Steamed string beans, okra and carrots if desired.
- Cup of alfalfa or mint tea.

MENU VII

Breakfast

- Tall glass of freshly squeezed orange or grapefruit juice.
- If you have orange juice, then have ½ grapefruit topped with honey.
- Old-fashioned rolled oats soaked overnight.
  Add ground almonds, pecans or filberts and 1 tablespoon wheat germ.
  Mix well before serving.
- Cup of rosemary, mint or camomile tea.

Lunch

- Large tomato stuffed with yogurt.
  Sprinkle with chopped nuts and wheat germ.
- Glass of soy, seed or nut milk.

Dinner

- Tall glass of fresh carrot or other vegetable juice.
- Mix well: shredded cabbage, grated carrots and chopped, minced or grated onions.
  Garnish with pumpkin, sunflower or sesame seeds.
  Top with one of the salad dressings.
- Cup of mint, alfalfa or other herb tea.

Note: These sample menus are intended to give you an idea of the ingredients involved and possible combinations. I want to urge you, however, to be creative. Experiment with the items. Make your own favorites. Especially if you have purchased new equipment—a blender, a juicer and a Kitchen Magician—use them as creative tools. Just remember that I urge you not to mix fruits and vegetables together in the same meal. Mixing fruit with vegetable juices, or vegetables with fruit juices, is all right. And especially be creative with seed garnishes. Get used to using sunflower seeds, sesame seeds and pumpkin seeds. In salads, use them as you ordinarily would grated cheese or hard-boiled egg.

As an addition to the weight-on diet, use natural vitamin supplements, iron tablets, multivitamins, vitamin E, protein powder, tablet or liquid. You may take flaxseed before meals. Also brewer's yeast. Dried beans or peas may also be used. And get used to drinking herb teas, peppermint, alfalfa, and the like, instead of coffee.

When I first started out in show business, it was an insult if the audience threw fruit or vegetables on the stage. Now I'd consider it a compliment! But before going further in the Dick Gregory Natural Diet, I want to drop in this very important suggestion for thoroughly cleaning fruits and vegetables. You want to remove all traces of sprays and poisons used to ward off "pests" in the orchards and fields. If you don't get rid of the traces of chemical sprays, those poisons just might regard your insides as one of the pests! So go to the drugstore and get some chemically pure *hydrochloric acid*. Simply place the fruit and vegetables, after they've been washed, in an earthenware pot filled with a 1 percent hydrochloric acid solution. That's 1 ounce of hydrochloric acid to 3 quarts of water. Keep the fruits and vegetables in the solution for about five minutes, then rinse and use. You can keep and use the solution for a week before making a fresh batch of spray remover.

Now I want to give you my two favorite blender/juicer recipes. These two treats alone will make it worth your while to get hold of a blender and juicer! One is a fruit soup, which I suppose I ought to dedicate to all those who've been keeping the war in Vietnam going, thereby keeping me on a liquid diet. The other is a fruit and nut mulch which will put the ice cream man out of business once you've tasted it. Both recipes are guaranteed to provide quick energy and pure nourishment to keep up your strength during human rights demonstrations, extended boycotts, and such.

DICK GREGORY'S NUTCRACKER SWEET

Juice up, in an electric or manually operated juicer, 3 pears, 3 apples, 6 oranges, 1 lemon, 2 grapefruits, about a pound of grapes (green, red and purple mixed) and a carton of strawberries. Remove from carton, of course. Mix the juices thoroughly in the blender. Get a large pitcher or some other large container. In the container place ¼ pound sesame seeds, ¼ pound sunflower seeds, ¼ pound almonds. Also put in some unsulfured dried fruit. You can get mixed dried fruit prepackaged. Or you can make your own mixture—dried apricots, figs, dates, raisins, peaches and prunes. Be sure the dates and prunes are pitted! A couple of small handfuls of dried fruit should do it. Pour the juice mixture over the nuts and dried fruit and let stand in the refrigerator overnight. At least several hours. Then put the whole business into the blender once again and blend it at high speed. Shut the blender off and you've got your nutcracker sweet. Sit down, relax, play a little Tchaikovsky and enjoy!

DICK GREGORY'S ALWAYS IN THE SOUP
HEALTH POWER UPLIFT

Cut up 2 tomatoes, 1 cucumber, 1 small squash, 1 bell pepper, 1 avocado. Put them in the blender with ½ small onion and a small clove of garlic. Add necessary pure water—1 or 2 cups. Add 2 tablespoons honey. Blend together thoroughly. It can be served cold. Or it can be simmered in a double boiler to be served warm. However you eat it, you'll be in the soup with me.

Now for the Dick Gregory Natural Diet for folks who want to lose weight or get themselves together with Mother Nature. This diet is not a quick-loss, fad diet. It's a suggestion for changing your eating habits for the rest of your life. Most folks eat everything from fruit to nuts anyway. My diet just skips the stuff in between. Weight loss will follow, of course. But more important than any weight considerations is the *nutritional* advantage. The Dick Gregory Natural Diet over the entire period combines changing to raw foods, detoxifying the body, fasting, eliminating meat, dairy and poultry products from the diet, and most important, I imagine, to most folks, doing all this over a period of four months rather than overnight.

The first month I'm recommending changing the first two meals. Fruit and fruit juice will be taken for breakfast and lunch. The evening meal will be what you always eat. Or the adventuresome folks might want to plunge right into a salad evening meal. The second month will continue fruit and fruit juice for the first two meals and a salad evening meal allowing the use of hard-boiled egg and grated cheese. The third month will be fruit juice the first two meals, salad for dinner, but now you'll replace the grated cheese and hard-boiled egg with seed garnishes—pumpkin, sunflower and sesame seeds.

Finally, during the fourth month, when you'll really be cleaning out the system, you'll have seven days of fruit, seven days of fruit juice, three days of only pure water, four days of fruit juice, and finally back to seven days of fruit. That's twenty-eight days, but don't put off starting the Dick Gregory Natural Diet until the fourth month falls in February. (It might be leap year, and then where would you be?) Because, after the final twenty-eight-day period, I hope you'll go back to the diet of the third month for the rest of your life.

THE DICK GREGORY NATURAL DIET

FIRST MONTH

Breakfast

Breakfast is the same for the whole month. The freshly squeezed juice of 2 grapefruits, 6 oranges and 2 lemons or limes. Sweeten with honey to taste.

Lunch

Lunches consist of only fresh fruits. Typical lunch menus would be:

MENU I

2 apples

2 pears

½ pound grapes

MENU II

1 banana

2 oranges

2 apples

MENU III

Your own!

Have fun combining fruits. Use berries and melons in season. Don't forget cherries, peaches, apricots, etc. Sweeten with honey, and do your fruit thing!

Dinner

The choice is up to you. If you want to hang on to those eating violations for another month, go ahead. You better save up to go to restaurants and lunch counters for the last time! And as long as you're choosing to continue to abuse your body, you may just as well have cocktails, dessert and coffee.

Or you may want to start right away with a large green salad for dinner—garnished with hard-boiled egg, grated cheese, your favorite salad dressing, whatever. Again, it's up to you if you want to cut out meat even as a salad garnish during this month.

SECOND MONTH

Breakfast

Same fruit juice combination as the first month: 2 freshly squeezed grapefruits, 6 oranges and 2 lemons or limes.

Lunch

By now you will probably have become such an expert at fruit combining that you will look forward to your fruit meal. Have you used tangerines yet? I hesitate to say it, but I hope you didn't forget about watermelon!

Dinner

Now you have to change that dinner menu, if you haven't done so already. Get out your Kitchen Magician, your chopper, shredder, sharp knife or grater and try some of these:

MENU I

Shred finely 1 cup each of green, white and red cabbage. Mix well with mayonnaise, or lemonaise, or lemon juice and honey, or herb dressing. You may garnish with a hard-boiled egg or two and some shredded cheese.

MENU II

One-half cup each of chopped cauliflower, carrots, asparagus and beets. Add 2 tablespoons chopped onion; ½ clove garlic, mashed; 2 tablespoons chopped parsley. Your favorite dressing, or lemon juice, olive oil and honey. You may garnish with grated cheese and one or two hard-boiled eggs, sliced or chopped.

MENU III

Two leaves of romaine lettuce or 10 leaves of Bibb lettuce. Cut up carrots, celery, radishes, parsley. Again add your grated cheese, hard-boiled egg, salad dressing.

MENU IV

Make a fruit salad. Start with soaked dried figs, dates, raisins. Add cubed apples, pineapple. Mix in a tablespoon of wheat germ, then a tablespoon or two of honey.

MENU V

Try this tasty combination: one avocado, six ripe pitted olives, one small cucumber, one medium to large tomato, one bell pepper. That's a fruit salad, believe it or not.

MENU VI

Make a kind of Waldorf salad with sliced apples, raisins, cubed pineapple and nuts (almonds, filberts, pecans). Mix with lemonaise, or lemon juice, honey and olive oil, or, during this month, mayonnaise if you prefer.

Don't forget in making up your salad creations that you can use raw spinach as a delightfully healthful ingredient.

During the first two months, if you are hungry in the evening you may have a half or two halves of a grapefruit with honey for sweetening. Also, during your evening salad meal, you can have two types of salad, menu V or VI with any of the other menus, as long as you wait a half hour to two hours before mixing the vegetable and fruit salads in your stomach.

THIRD MONTH

Breakfast and *lunch* follow the same pattern as the first two months. Did you lose weight last month? How do you feel? Remember that old Alka-Seltzer commercial where the guy talks to his stomach? I'll bet you and your stomach are on better speaking terms now. Just wait! Your whole system is going to *love* you.

Dinner will continue with fresh raw salad, but now you're cutting out the hard-boiled egg and cheese garnishes and the mayonnaise, and replacing them with seed garnishes and one of the natural salad dressings.

The seed garnishes would be ¼ cup sunflower seeds, ¼ cup pumpkin seeds or ¼ cup sesame seeds; ¼ cup flaked, chopped or ground almonds.

Use the salad menus from the second month, or those you have developed yourself, *but no cheese, mayonnaise or hard-boiled egg.* Add ¼ teaspoon or so of kelp if you can get hold of it.

If you get hungry in the evening during this month, soaked

dried fruit with honey should be used to assuage that late-evening appetite.

FOURTH MONTH

The real cleansing begins this month. The *first seven days* eat only fruit, three meals a day. You can also drink a tall glass of fresh fruit juice before each meal. Use a single fruit juice—orange, grapefruit, freshly squeezed, apple made in your juicer, or pear, or whatever. Dilute the juice made in your juicer somewhat with distilled water or spring water, as much as half for grape and apple juices; let your taste be your guide. You can also use the freshly squeezed combination of juices you have been using. Of course, those juices can always be sweetened with honey.

For this seven-day period you will be making a three-meal-a-day habit of the same kind of fare you have been taking for lunches. Remember, you can include tomatoes and cucumbers as fruits. And don't forget things like avocado, papaya and tropical fruits.

The *second seven days* take only fruit juice. I hope by now you do have a juicer so you won't just have to take freshly squeezed juice. Remember to dilute with pure or distilled water the stronger juices you make. Drink an eight-ounce glass of juice every time you feel hunger. If you leave the house, take a large thermos of juice with you. Or take a flask and have fun with folks by admitting you're on the juice.

After the seven days of fruit juice, you are ready to put your body on a fast. For the next *three days,* take only pure water. Every time you feel hunger, drink your water. Try to drink a gallon each day. In planning your activities during the day, don't forget your increased need for "comfort."

After three days of only water, go back to *four more days* of fruit juice, followed by *seven days* of fruit.

I want to emphasize again the importance of taking enemas to help flush out the poisons and waste your body will be getting rid of during this four-month period. During the first two months you should take a weekly enema. The second month you could begin to take an enema every third day. The third month should definitely begin the every-third-day pattern. During the fourth month take an enema every other day, or every day.

That's the Dick Gregory Natural Diet for Folks Who Eat. It comes to you straight from the kitchens of Mother Nature—with a little help from her friends: a juicer, a blender, a piece of muslin cloth and hydrochloric acid.

Try it and I'll make you one guarantee. For the first time in your life you'll feel *really* clean!

10

Mother Nature's Mothers— and Their Offspring

In his marvelous little booklet, *Your Vegetarian Baby*, Dr. Pietro Rotondi reminds: "Women and Mothers of today have the power to save mankind from further trouble, future wars, pestilence and disease, and to redeem man to his rightful place on earth, especially in relation to his Maker. The Mother-to-be should at all times remember her high calling fearlessly, and with great joy await her time of fulfillment."

How well are mothers of America following Dr. Rotondi's advice? Well, according to a *New York Times* article by Nadine Brozan on August 30, 1972, the Gerber's baby food company figures that every baby in America has consumed seventy-two dozen jars of their product by the time the infant switches to an adult menu at about one and a half years old! That's 864 times a baby has to get used to the processed food habit, to say nothing of the meat and overcooking habit, before the tot is eighteen months old. And that's just one brand.

The commercial baby food industry has been called on the carpet many times. A couple of years ago, Ralph Nader was condemning the practices of overcharging, adding MSG and using salt, sugar and starch in the preparation process. Even the National Academy of Sciences went along with removing MSG, since its sole purpose was to titillate the taste buds. But the Academy would not come out and say it was harmful. It also suggested salt levels should be reduced.

The point of all this is to illustrate how early in life we become accustomed to and learn to crave the inadequate junk diet from the supermarket shelf. As Dr. Rotondi says, mothers have it in their power to start children off right in their lifelong dietary pattern. If the mother doesn't teach the child to eat wrong, the child will have much less chance of ending up doing it!

Personally I have a double reason for not purchasing the popular commercial baby food. I reject both the processing and the advertising. On every tiny jar of Gerber's baby food, you will find a picture of a little smiling *white* baby! It may not seem so important on the surface, but can you imagine the effect that has on the developing young mind of a little *black* baby? A little black baby being fed from the Gerber's jar learns—even before she or he can walk or talk—to identify that smiling white baby with *food*. The unspoken message to the little black baby is that to get the basic sustenance of life you've got to go through white folks.

The best preparation for motherhood a mother-to-be can make is to vow to try to be a reflection of the Supreme Mother of all— Mother Nature. Thus the new mother-to-be will look to Mother Nature's design of proper planting for a clue in planning her own parenthood. In the order of nature, it is extremely important to plant seeds in the proper season. The conditions of the soil and the climate for growth will determine the quality of the crop. Seeds planted "out of time" yield an undesirable harvest.

It is the same with Mother Nature's mothers and fathers and

their offspring. The child should first be conceived in the minds of the mother and father and the proper climate should be established in the home. The condition of the bodies of the parents is very important to the growth and development of the new life they are planning to bring into the world, just as the condition of the soil determines the growth of the seedling.

Both mother and father should adopt a diet of feeding themselves upon life rather than death. They should practice a diet which is based upon Mother Nature's kingdoms of nutrition. There are three orders of growth among the living foods Mother Nature provides. The highest order consists of all things that grow on trees, nearest to the direct "cooking" of Mother Nature's sun— fruits, nuts, avocados. Next comes the intermediate level, those things which grow above the ground, yet very close to the earth— green leafy vegetables, tomatoes, legumes, some berries, grapes, herbs. Finally, there is Mother Nature's underground, all things which grow hidden in the earth—roots and tubers.

Mother Nature's "budding" parents should combine the kingdoms of nutrition, starting their day with a breakfast of fruit, fruit juice and nuts; taking fresh raw leafy vegetables and salads seasoned with natural herbs and seeds at midday; and including the root vegetables and their juices at the evening meal. They should spurn coffee, commercial tea, candy, tobacco and alcohol. Natural herb teas should replace coffee or commercial tea—red clover, alfalfa-mint, Golden Seal, camomile or sassafras. Only when the prospective new parents feel the "soil" of their bodies is ready should copulation for conception take place.

After the seed has been planted the new mother-to-be should drink ample supplies of raw fresh carrot juice, especially during the last three months. The vitamin A is so necessary for growth and carrot juice is also a rich source of calcium. One pint of carrot juice daily has more constructive body value than *25 pounds* of calcium tablets. Nursing mothers will also find that the quality of their milk is improved by cultivating the carrot juice habit.

Mothers-to-be should begin a practice they will later pass on to their children—namely, avoiding the use of cow's milk. As K. Morishita has pointed out in his essay *Nutrition and Physiology of Milk:* ". . . human milk contains phosphorus [as opposed to the great amount of calcium found in cow's milk]. This element is very important for brain growth and development. The human baby develops its brain first, while the animal develops its bone structure first. Therefore, milk for a human and for that of an animal naturally should be different. Giving cow's milk to the human infant, without thinking about such an order of nature, is too simple-minded." Expectant mothers should begin making and using soy milk or nut milk or sesame seed milk, a practice they would continue after their child is born.

Milk is the perfect food for Mother Nature's babies *only* if it is mother's milk. If babies are bottle fed they should only have Mother Nature's milk—soy, seed or nut milk—the milk intended for *human* baby consumption. The baby nursed by its mother may be given raw fruit and vegetable juices between nursing periods after two months. The fruits and vegetables must be fully ripened, and the juice must be extracted fresh for each feeding.

As an alternate to raw fruit and vegetable juices between feedings, alfalfa-mint, camomile, alfalfa or oat straw tea may be given with unpasteurized honey added. Mother Nature's mothers should get their babies in the honey habit as quickly as other mothers get them in the meat habit. A teaspoon of raw honey added to a cup of water may be started at birth in preference to plain water. (Most health experts today advise parents to avoid introducing honey until the child is one to avoid the risk of infant botulism. —Ed.)

When the baby can masticate well, the slow feeding of solid foods can begin. As soon as possible, start the child on raw fruit and vegetable eating. Fully ripe mashed tomato may be offered to a baby as early as eight weeks old, provided it is no more than a teaspoonful. Be sure that all fruits are *fully* ripe. Early solid food offerings may be mashed fully ripe banana, or apples and avocado. Peel and grate apple pulp and heat slightly if desired. Mash avocado and add just a few drops of lemon, lime or tomato juice (fresh, of course). Fresh peeled tomato may be pushed through a sieve and served plain or topped with avocado. A liberal sprinkling of fresh parsley juice may also be added.

The blender is an invaluable aid in the initial raw food preparations. Some suggested blender formulas follow.

Natural Blender Formulas for the Growing Baby

All vegetables should be slightly steamed, not boiled or cooked, in a stainless steel waterless cooker. Use the blender to liquefy all solids and strain.

Formula 1	
Soy, nut or seed milk	5 ounces
Carrots	19
Pure water	4
	28 ounces

Formula 2	
Soy, nut or seed milk	12 ounces
Carrots	19
Almonds, soaked and skinned	1
Water	7
	39 ounces

Formula 3	
Soy, nut or seed milk	5 ounces
Figs, dried and soaked	3
Brazil nuts	1
Water	32
	41 ounces

Formula 4	
Soy, nut or seed milk	12 ounces
Dates, dried and soaked	2
Almonds, soaked and skinned	1
Water	24
	39 ounces

Formula 5	
Soy, nut or seed milk	2 ounces
Almonds, soaked and skinned	1
Carrots	19
Water	18
	40 ounces

Formula 6	
Almonds, soaked and skinned	2 ounces
Celery	2
Carrots	10
Lettuce	2
Water	28
	44 ounces

Formula 7	
Beets	7 ounces
Carrots	13
Soy, nut or seed milk	6
Water	8
	34 ounces

Formula 8	
Coconut, fresh	1 ounce
Apples	19
Banana	4
Soy, nut or seed milk	6
Water	10
	40 ounces

Formula 9	
Avocado	4 ounces
Papaya	9
Soy, nut or seed milk	12
Water	3
	28 ounces

Mother Nature's parents should be able to afford a blender out of what they save in doctor bills alone. But there are other savings natural parents will have because they will be clothing and caring for their infant as Mother Nature intends and not as fashion and social expectation dictate.

Let me illustrate. The baby who belongs to Mother Nature should not wear shoes. Cotton booties will do fine. The baby should have freedom of movement. The soles of the feet are one of Mother Nature's greatest eliminators of body poisons. That is why walking barefoot in Mother Nature's grass, sand or earth is so beneficial. When a person walks barefoot, the nervous system is literally grounded to the earth. The nerve endings in the soles of the feet are in physical contact with the source of life and growth.

When the baby begins to walk, sandals are the most natural foot covering to allow for the strengthening of the foot and ankle and also to maintain correct posture. The more porous fabrics, like cotton and cotton flannel, are preferable to the warmth and confinement of wool. And when it comes to toiletries, Mother Nature's babies need only two items: Epsom salts for bathing and olive oil for the skin.

The Bible reminds us that "the sins of the fathers shall be visited upon the third and fourth generations." Without getting into a discussion of theology, I do know that sin is equivalent to disobedience. And certainly humankind has been disobedient to Mother Nature for quite a few generations. The tragedy is that the sin is passed on—*taught*—to generation after generation.

Fathers and mothers of one generation, perhaps this very one, have the opportunity to change the course. It is so simple. Don't start *your* children on the course of disobedience. If they don't learn from you, they probably never will.

11

Dick Gregory's Questions and Answers for Folks with Special Problems and Interests Who Eat

Q. *Mr. Gregory, you were a track star in high school and college. I'm an athlete myself. What kind of diet do you recommend for me?*
A. I'm glad you asked that, son. But would you stop running in place while I'm talking to you? The first thing I would say is no meat! Remember what I've already said about meat forming uric acid and the crystals collecting in the muscles. No athlete can afford to have that happen. It's the best way to become a spectator!

Besides, the proteins available from raw foods—fruits, vegetables, seeds and nuts—are superior to meat protein. I know of studies which prove athletes have improved their performance by changing from a 100-gram-a-day animal protein diet to a 50-gram-a-day natural food protein diet. Natural carbohydrates and protein are what you need.

Get used to eating sunflower seeds, sesame seeds and pumpkin seeds. Don't ever snack on candies, drink soft drinks or eat pastries. Of course, cut out coffee, alcohol and tobacco. You can drink natural herb teas—alfalfa, peppermint, basil, rosemary, and the like. Take a little pure honey for that quick energy, when everybody else is eating candy bars or sugar. See what happens. You might get a gold medal. Or even five!

Eat as few different kinds of foods as possible at any one meal. Eat fruit and vegetables at separate meals. And eat high-protein foods first when they are eaten with other foods.

Q. *Mr. Gregory, I'm past the age of being trusted—you know, thirty and all that. My question is—uh, well, I don't quite know how to ask it. I'm worried about losing my power, or my ability to perform. Do you know what I mean?*

A. Yes, I think I do. Well, to protect and stimulate your glands I'd recommend wheat germ, brewer's yeast, pure honey, sesame, sunflower and pumpkin seeds, and sarsaparilla tea. Drink sarsaparilla at least twice a day. I guess the old cowboys must have known something. Maybe sarsaparilla also improves your aim!

Pay special attention to your colon and the process of elimination. Fresh fruits and fruit juices will help. Have a thorough cleaning out with high enemas or colonic irrigations. Get a juicer and drink a lot of carrot and spinach juices—10 ounces carrot to 6 ounces spinach.

Stay away from all foods with chemical additives. Take some natural vitamin E supplements. You'll also get vitamin E from spinach, lettuce and watercress. Cut your salt intake down to a bare minimum, or cut it out entirely. If you are eating primarily or exclusively raw fruits and vegetables, you won't need the salt.

Q. *Mr. Gregory, I have these very close veins. . . .*

A. That's varicose, ma'am.

Q. *That's what I said.* Very *close. They're very close to poppin' through my stockings. Can you help me?*

A. There's not much I can do, but you can help yourself by eliminating all fried foods, starches, sandwiches, pastries, pie, cake, and the like from your diet starting now. Drink at least two or three pints of fresh fruit or vegetable juice each day.

I'd really recommend a fast, but at least change your diet to raw salads and raw fruits. Cut salt out of your diet. And I'd also advise you to get some kelp food supplement from a health food store and take it each day.

Q. *Mr. Gregory, my grandma's got terrible swollen ankles. What should I tell her to do?*

A. It sounds like your grandma needs a good detoxifying. She probably eats starches and fried food. Tell her to stop. If she drinks coffee, she should cut it out. Not only the coffee, but the white sugar I'm sure she puts in it, to say nothing of cream, is bad for her. Tell her to replace that coffee with ginseng tea.

Let's face it. Grandma is getting into her ripe years. So she should be eating more and more *ripe* fruit. And drinking juices. The digestive process is slowing down and she needs foods the body can handle more easily. It wouldn't hurt at all for her to take some natural vitamin C supplement.

To sum it all up, my advice is to "get fresh" with grandma. Tell her to eat fresh raw foods.

Q. *Mr. Gregory, as you can see, I've developed quite a "bay window."* . . .

A. I see you've lost quite a bit of hair too. Unless that's a skin wig.

Q. *What am I supposed to do?*

A. I'll give it to you straight from the hip; excuse me, that was a bad analogy. Take enemas! You too are suffering from toxemia.

You've got impacted waste matter in the colon which must come out. You've got a bloated stomach now, but if those toxic poisons stay in your system, you'll have a whole host of other troubles later on.

I notice you are smoking a cigarette. Stop that right now!

Q. *I've tried but . . .*

A. Well, be like Avis and try harder. No wonder you're full of poisons. Tobacco smoke contains two particularly irritating and vicious poisons—nicotine and acrolein. Inhaling tobacco smoke stimulates an excessive secretion of adrenaline. Look at the towel a heavy cigarette smoker uses when coming out of a steam bath. I mean *after* it has been used. The towel will be saturated with a perspiration residue that runs from tan to dark brown in color. And unless the steam bather happened to be Al Jolson in "blackface," the dark-colored residue is nicotine and acrolein coming out through the pores of the skin.

I'll bet you drink too.

Q. *Well, I take a nip now and then—but only after work.*

A. You mean *your* work. What about your body's work? Alcohol is devastating because it acts as a solvent for elements in the body which are only soluble in alcohol. It destroys the texture of the kidneys, hardens the liver and messes up the nerves closely related to the brain. So it eventually destroys the normal functions of observation, locomotion and concentration.

Q. *I'm sorry, what did you say? I was thinking about something else.*

A. I said, "concentration." If you drink you won't be able to concentrate.

Q. *Well, I guess I'll switch to soft drinks. And I'll eat candy to kill my urge for cigarettes.*

A. Ever hear the phrase "Jumping from the frying pan into the fire"? That's just what you'll be doing with that remedy.

It won't do any good to cut out booze and replace it with candy. Or soft drinks either. Both candy and soft drinks contain sugar. What happens when you cut the bar loose and pick up the candy-bar? Sugar in any form, candy or soft drinks, ferments in the system, forming *acetic acid, carbonic acid* and *alcohol.* So you're right back to booze!

Acetic acid is pretty powerful stuff. Ever had warts? Acetic acid is used to burn warts off the skin. I'll leave it to your imagination to figure out what it does to the intestines.

Drinking soft drinks or taking in sugar in any form overworks the pancreas. I'm talking, of course, about refined sugar, or commercial sugar. All sugar that has been processed with heat. I do not mean honey, date sugar, raw sugar, or any other natural sweetening.

Refined sugar is a "dead" processed product. It can be said it is a drug in the system. Folks who use too much sugar eventually go through the same internal bodily degeneration as a drug addict, or "junkie."

White sugar is worst of all, by the way, because it has been "refined" with sulfuric acid. And it steals calcium from the system.

Q. *Mr. Gregory, I've got two questions. What about salt? And should I take vitamins?*
A. I've got two answers. It's bad. And if you eat the right raw foods, you don't need 'em.

The body fluids contain 0.85 percent of salt. The percentage is maintained in the blood of all *healthy* folks. A radical change— excuse me, an extreme change . . . maybe I better say substantial change so there won't be any political overtones—a substantial change in the salt proportion causes serious changes in the blood elements.

Common table salt is another drug. It is the chemical combination of the soft, lustrous, silverlike metal sodium with the greenish yellow acrid poisonous gas chlorine. To this is often added another drug, potassium iodide, supposedly to give iodine.

When a change in the sodium balance occurs, too much table salt, in other words, a change in the water balance also results. Tissue spaces become waterlogged. Fluids gather in unaccustomed places. Swelling, in other words. Organs are swollen all out of proportion and their functions are interfered with; a vicious cycle of degeneration sets in. All organs and all body tissues will eventually be involved if proper balance is not restored.

All living matter contains salt. Therefore, if you consume the right kind of raw foods, your salt and mineral supply is taken care of. And for the iodine, kelp is the best possible source you can find. Use powdered kelp as a salt substitute and you will be doing your body a great favor.

Q. *Remember, Mr. Gregory, I also asked about vitamins.*

A. Oh, yes! Well, the same thing is true of vitamins. If you are really following a proper raw food diet, you will be getting all the vitamins you need. However, you can use vitamins you get from your health food store and some drugstores. Just be careful to look at the labels, read the contents, and be sure they are *natural* food supplements and not *chemical* food supplements. Your body can't use the chemicals.

While I am on the subject of supplements, let me mention the enzyme preparations available at the health food store. I hesitate to do it because it is like "cheating" on a truly proper diet. The various enzyme preparations are composed of enzymes active in the process of converting and absorbing nutrients in the alimentary canal. For example, there is amylase, which converts starch into sugar, papain, derived from the papaya, which converts protein into amino acids, and pancreatin, which contains four principle digestive enzymes. There are also preparations containing acids, like taurocholic acid and glutamic acid, which help digestion. Enzyme preparations are available in both tablet and chewing gum form.

The problem with enzyme preparations and all other vitamin supplements is that they allow you to continue to make violations in your eating habits and still get by. Health food stores are unfortunately in danger of becoming like the good, slick lawyers who get rich folks off the hook in court. They know their client is guilty, but they also know the loopholes to get the client off.

There should be no substitute for proper eating habits. At best vitamins should only be used as supplements to a raw, natural fruit and vegetable and nut and seed and some cereals diet.

With enzyme preparations, you can go to the restaurant and get by with ordering what you want if you pop some enzyme pills into your mouth before and after the meal and between courses. I've heard some health food authorities advise this. From my point of view, it is no substitute for cutting out restaurants entirely and getting back on good terms with Mother Nature.

Q. *Mr. Gregory, I've listened to all you said about sugar, soft drinks, candy, pastries and all those usual after-school snacks. But I've got some kids with a sweet tooth. They're going to eat something when they come home from school. What should I do?*

A. Do you have a blender?

Q. *No.*

A. Then run to the nearest Sears, Roebuck store and get one. And while you're there, pick up one of those fantastically reasonably priced juicers. I really can't give Sears enough credit for putting these two very important items in the price range of most folks. At

Sears you can get a juicer and blender for the price saved on cutting out tobacco and alcohol alone! To say nothing of candy and soft drinks. Of course, you'll also find a variety of juicers available at health food stores at many different prices.

Pardon the digression. Let me give you some blender recipes which you can fix for your kids, or if the kids are old enough, teach them to fix for themselves. The same as they would a peanut butter sandwich.

PRUNE NUT SNACK OR DESSERT

Soak large prunes in a Mason jar filled with pure cold water in the refrigerator overnight. Make sure the top is tightly screwed on. Next morning remove the pits from the prunes. Chop or finely mash nuts—almonds or filberts—in a nut grinder or blender. Mix the ground nuts with sesame seeds and honey. Stuff the prunes with this mixture. And there's a snack better than any candy bar!

STUFFED DATE SNACK OR DESSERT

For a variation, stuff pitted dates with the ground nut and honey mixture. Roll the dates in shredded coconut. Keep under refrigeration until ready to serve.

APRICOT BUTTER

Soak 2 cups of dried, unsulfured apricots in 2 cups of water in a Mason jar overnight. Screw the top on tightly. The next day, put it all in a blender, liquid and apricots, and add the juice of one lemon and ½ cup honey. Blend and put back in the jar. Some people use it on whole wheat bread or toast, but I would eat it as a pudding.

BANANA NUT ROLL

Grind almonds, pecans or filberts in a blender or nut grinder. Peel and halve bananas. Roll each banana half in the nuts. And you have a nutty Chiquita Banana delight!

BLENDER FRUIT BOWL

Mix 1 cup chopped figs, 1 cup dates, 1 cup raisins and 1 cup coconut milk or other nut milk. Add 1 tablespoon lemon juice. Blend thoroughly and serve in bowls.

Above all, keep plenty of fresh ripe fruit on hand for your kids to eat. They will soon lose their taste for candy. And remember to keep melons in the refrigerator. They are excellent appetite pleasers!

Q. *One final question, Mr. Gregory. You mentioned natural sweetening in preference over sugar, especially honey. What about people who have diabetes?*
A. I'm really glad you asked about that, honey. I mean I'm glad you asked about that *honey.* It is very, very important that anyone suffering from diabetes use only *tupelo* honey. It is available at the health food store and is the *only* kind of honey diabetics should touch!

12

Dick Gregory's Natural Diet for Pets and Plants Who Eat

This chapter is fondly dedicated to Quasimodo, Mississippi, and J. Edgar Churchill, who live in the household of Sandy and Mary Jo Baron.

Readers who have got this far along in the *Natural Diet* should also be concerned about other living things they bring into their homes—namely pets and plants. Since dogs and cats are the most common household pets, we'll focus primarily on their dietary needs.

The problems for pets begin when they leave Mother Nature and enter so-called civilized households. In their natural state, pets would live according to Mother Nature's rules, in sickness and in health, getting the proper diet, the right amount of exercise, air and sunlight.

When pets enter the average household, they can't see the forest or the trees, and they become dependent upon their "masters" rather than Mother Nature. And, like their owners, pets have poor health almost from birth. Dogs, for example, are brought into an urban environment with its polluted air and treated water; cooped up all day in an overcrowded apartment; fed from the processed food shelf of their owner's favorite supermarket; and, when they do get outside in the open spaces for a few moments, forced to accept the degrading substitute of a fire hydrant instead of an oak tree! It's little wonder that household pets are found suffering from all the ailments known to the human beings that keep them—from eczema to nephritis, from diabetes to cancer, from rheumatism to heart failure.

Mother Nature never lets go completely. No matter how domesticated dogs and cats become, or how fat, lazy and out of shape their owners encourage them to be, the "call of the wild" can still be detected in the simplest mannerisms of household pets. The fierce beauty and mystery of a cat's eyes and the swift, silent grace of its movements are a constant reminder that the cat is the distant cousin of the lion and the tiger. And a dog's kinship to the wolf is seen in its natural inclination to chase and hunt, or its tendency to turn around before lying down for a nap, just as its ancestors did to trample out a grassy spot in the wilderness to provide protection from a potential enemy.

No matter how "well cared for" by its owner, a dog will still follow its ancestral tradition of burying a bone to provide for future needs. And even though barking is a trait only of domesticated dogs (wild dogs howl and sometimes yelp but never bark), little Rover will often howl on moonlit nights, calling the hunting pack as his great-great-grandparents did many generations ago.

People are funny about their pets and their pets' diet. When you suggest to some folks that they ought to try putting their dogs and cats on a meatless diet, they will respond as though their little pets had never been domesticated! They will say, "Dogs and cats are supposed to eat meat. After all, they're descended from tigers and wolves!" Of course, if there was any real practicing line of descent, the chances are the pets would already have consumed their owners and their owners' kids!

Sometimes a pet owner will rationalize, "I tried giving my pet fruits and vegetables and more natural foods, but it preferred the canned pet food." It never seems to occur to the pet owner that the dog would prefer to relieve itself on the carpet, and would probably prefer *not* to roll over and play dead! Pet owners think nothing of housebreaking a dog, or training it to do tricks or to attack unwanted visitors; in short, to do things for the *owner's* benefit. But the same owner resists changing a pet's diet for the *pet's* benefit, and training the pet to eat it!

It is true that dogs and cats, in their most natural state, are carnivores, or meat-eaters. Just as human beings in their most natural state are fruit-eaters! But humans have adapted themselves to eating meat, and dogs and cats *can* adapt themselves to *not* eating meat. Actually, a natural diet for dogs and cats would include meat, but never *cooked* meat or any cooked food.

The pet dog begging under the family dinner table learns to eat the entire "mess" his owners devour—rich gravies, mashed potatoes, fried steak, sweet rolls, desserts, or whatever. To make matters worse, the dog gulps or bolts its food, rather than chewing it, so it does not get the benefit of insalivating the food in the mouth to start the digestive process.

Dogs and cats fed from the pet food shelf of the supermarket learn to eat denatured foods, the residues of meats, cereals and the like, after all the healthful nutrients have been removed and harmful chemical additives and preservatives put in. The entire concoction has been cooked to death so that it may be kept on the supermarket shelf indefinitely. It is little wonder that "finicky Morris" in the television cat food commercial turns up his nose at so many of his owner's offerings! He wants to hang on to at least *one* of his nine lives.

Until they passed the devitalizing habit on to their beloved pets, humans were the only creatures in the world that ate their food cooked. You'd never find a gorilla frying up some bananas for dinner or a lion charcoal-broiling a zebra steak. Cats don't often run to the oven with a mouse or bird they've captured, and a dog wouldn't naturally prepare its rabbit dinner in a stew.

It is little wonder then that the main cause of sickness in household pets is a form of toxemia, resulting from improper eating habits and the inability of the animal to rid its body of toxic waste. A diet of "people food for pets," in the form of either table leftovers or canned processed foods, is sometimes too much for an animal to bear. People eat so-called enriched white bread, in which the heat applied destroys the vitamin E among other things. Feed that to a dog for nine straight days and the dog will die. But before dying, the dog will go stark, raving mad, developing what veterinarians call "running fits."

Although raw meat is part of the natural diet of dogs and cats, it is by no means the only item on a proper pet menu, or even the largest proportional item, and dogs and cats fed wholly upon fat and meat would become round and plump, but would die of starvation. Pets given a balanced nonmeat diet would survive quite well.

Let me just say a further word about the raw meat used in a pet's diet. Some pet owners, who would object to the killing of animals for the human diet, justify their purchasing meat from the butcher for their pets' consumption because the pets are natural carnivores. So they feed their pets beef, horse meat, pork, lamb, liver and all other forms of butchershop raw meat. But that is not the *natural* raw meat diet of the carnivorous pet! To be consistent, such a pet owner would feed a dog raw rabbit, or chicken, or any of the small animals or birds the pet would naturally seize as prey. If I were a pet owner, my own personal conviction would demand that my pet get its source of protein from nonflesh sources. Once a pet is taken into the home, it is not living in its ancestral natural environment anyway, and my reading and conversations have convinced me that a pet could live quite healthily on a balanced nonflesh diet.

A balanced diet for dogs and cats is not unlike that for humans. Therefore the suggestions of the Natural Diet for Folks Who Eat are applicable to pets. Fruits are valuable in pet diets, since they are rich in alkaline minerals and vitamins and organic acids and help to neutralize toxic acids and wastes. Dogs and cats will learn to enjoy the pulp of peaches, pears, plums, apples, avocados, bananas, watermelons, tomatoes and, of course, grapes. The Song of Solomon in the Bible, chapter 2, verse 15, reminds us that the dog's ancestral cousins had a fondness for grapes: "Take us the foxes, the little foxes, that spoil the vines; for our vines have tender grapes." Tropical fruits like mangoes, avocados and papayas are excellent food for all pets, and smaller breeds of dogs should especially be trained to eat them regularly.

Fats and oils, contained in such foods as avocados, olives, nuts, soybeans, cheese, etc., will help prevent dryness, scaliness and inflammation of the skin, growth failures, kidney and liver ailments in pets. Some dogs can eat whole nuts as they come from the shell, but it is usually best to grind them in a grinder and serve them raw with chopped or grated vegetables—carrots, string beans, turnip greens and other leafy vegetables.

Three teaspoons of olive oil, soy oil or some nut oil should be mixed in the food of dogs each week, and cats should receive one teaspoonful weekly.

Carbohydrate foods such as squash, corn, potatoes, carrots, beans, grains and peas are good for pets. And foods rich in minerals are also necessary: fresh leafy vegetables and fruits, celery, lettuce, collards, spinach, parsley, mustard, turnip tops, cabbage, potatoes, melons, berries, apples, figs, pears and grapes. Other rich mineral sources are watercress, dill, turnip leaves, savoy cabbage, kale, lettuce, dandelion, Swiss chard, okra, tomatoes, berries, citrus fruits and nuts.

Chopped vegetables, leaves and herbs can be added to the meat in serving pet meals. Any seaweed product—especially kelp—is also an excellent addition to meat servings. But *cereal should never be mixed with meat* (as is done in processed pet foods) because the combination can cause a great deal of fermentation in the pet's stomach, resulting in an uncomfortable, bloated feeling and foul breath.

The ideal cereal food for pets is in the flaked form such as oat flakes, wheat flakes, barley flakes or rye flakes. If you have a health food store in your community, you will find a full selection of top quality cereal foods which contain a variety of whole grains.

Remember that cereal is hard for the pet to digest, unless it is *slightly* cooked, or "predigested," in the form the natural carnivore would get it. The natural meat-eating animal would begin by eating the stomach contents of the small herb- and grain-eating prey it had killed for food. Thus the cereal would already be partially digested. Cereals used for pet food can also be soaked in raw milk, soy milk or vegetable broth to make it more digestible.

If the pet has a sweet tooth to be satisfied, avoid synthetic sweets and candies. Instead, grind a few figs, dates and raisins in a meat grinder, forming the ground-out goodies into little balls. These can be fed as a complete meal. And be sure to purchase unsulfured fruits when buying dried fruits, as sulfur dioxide and sulfurous acid interfere with the function of the kidneys.

Meat should not constitute more than 25 percent of the pet's diet. If the pet is getting top quality protein in the rest of its diet, 10 to 15 percent meat consumption is quite adequate. Cereals should comprise about 25 or 30 percent of the diet and honey should be added to the cereal mixture. Meat and cereals should *never* be given at the same feeding.

The major portion of the diet should consist of the chopped or grated vegetables, ground nuts, honey, fruits, fresh or dried, raw milk, soybeans and soybean milk (made by adding five cups of water to a cup of soybean flour), cheese and other raw natural foods. Once the pet has become accustomed to eating the natural nonflesh sources of protein, I would strongly urge cutting down meat consumption to a bare minimum.

Undoubtedly, many pets that are used to eating processed foods, table scraps, pasteurized milk and commercially prepared pet "treats" will not show immediate enthusiasm for the new natural foods. Rather than "biting the hand that feeds them"—as they would be justified in doing!—pets resign themselves to the "garbage" diet of their owners. The owner must "own up" to the responsibility for having swayed the pet away from its natural dietary inclinations in the first place and take on the new responsibility of *training* the pet in a new diet.

The easiest way would be to place the pet on a liquid diet for three days—like one bowl of raw milk daily or a broth or slightly warmed juice. Then, to break the liquid diet, offer the pet a baked potato, mixed with chopped leafy vegetables or grated carrot. Or break the liquid diet with a slightly steamed whole-grain dish, with honey and squash mixed in.

Owners shouldn't be upset when their pets refuse food, especially their cats. In a natural state, it's not unusual for carnivores to eat only two or three times a week. When a cat refuses to eat food that is offered, it does not necessarily mean the cat doesn't like the offering. The cat just might not be hungry. The food should be left for fifteen minutes, then removed and offered fresh the same time the next day, or six hours later. If the food is wholesome and the cat is hungry, the pet will eat.

Like their owners, pets benefit from fasting. Remember that an animal in its natural state will abstain from food whenever it feels out of sorts. Only owners push food in a sick animal's face! Putting a pet on a fast regularly, as part of the diet pattern, a minimum of two days a month, and preferably one day a week for adult pets, will help keep weight down; health, vitality and happiness up; and accumulated toxic waste out. Pets with higher amounts of raw meat in their diet should definitely follow the one-day-a-week fasting pattern. Pets have been known to benefit from fasting when they are ill. Give the pet only pure water until the symptoms begin to subside, and then provide only fruit juice or broth.

Pure water, sunlight, air, rest and exercise are also important ingredients in the Natural Diet for Pets Who Eat. Animals in their natural state will go miles to find water that suits their taste. Distilled water and rain or spring water is best for pets. It should be provided fresh in a clean container. Dirt and scum allowed to accumulate in the drinking bowl of the pet will discourage its drinking the proper amounts of water. As with humans, it is best for pets not to drink water with their meals. Owners should remove the water container an hour before food is given and replace it two hours later. Tap water should be avoided if possible, but if tap water is used, it should be boiled first.

Growing pets should be placed in the morning and evening

sunlight for at least half-hour periods each day. A sick animal should be kept in a room which is well ventilated and exposed to the sunlight. Pets should be encouraged to exercise, as they often live the easy and lazy life of their owners. Train your pet to play, to retrieve sticks and balls, and set aside a half hour to an hour each day to engage your pet in this exercise activity.

Owners who give their pets a raw food diet, pure water, fresh air, regular periods in the sunlight and proper exercise are indeed an "animal's best friend.

Frequency of Feeding

Puppies and kittens need more frequent feeding—four times a day. Adult animals, ten months and beyond, need feeding less frequently—no more than twice a day—and adult dogs and cats can both do well on once-a-day meals.

Puppies from weaning to the age of five months may be fed at regular five-hour intervals—8 A.M., 1 P.M., and 11 P.M.—except for Sunday, when all food should be withheld until 1 P.M. From five to ten months, they may receive twice-a-day feedings—1 P.M. and between 6 and 8 P.M.—and only the evening meal on Sunday. After ten months, adult dogs should either follow the same feeding pattern as the five-to-eight-month animals or be reduced to one meal a day. One day a week, adult animals should be fasted, given only pure water for their diet.

The same pattern may be followed for kittens and cats, cutting feeding down to three times a day, or even two times a day, after the age of seven months. After ten months, the adult feeding pattern may be fixed—twice a day or once a day—remembering the fasting day and also the fact that cats have more of a tendency to do their own dietary thing of eating only when hungry.

Amount to Feed

It is difficult to prescribe the exact amount of food to give a dog or cat. Pet owners will have to establish that for themselves, and, of course, for their pets. The amount of food varies with the breed and size of the pet, the amount of exercise it gets, and so on. For cats, if the proper weight is maintained and the pet remains playful and active, the food intake is probably correct. If the cat puts on weight, gets sluggish and perhaps even leaves food in the plate consistently, it's a clear sign pet owners are acting like parents and being overindulgent in the amount of food offered.

A starting point for establishing a dog's food intake according to the pet's size and weight would be:

Weight of Pet	Amount of Daily Food Intake
5 pounds	1 cup (8 ounces)
15	2 cups (16 ounces or 1 pound)
30	3 to 4 cups (1 to 1½ pounds)
50	5 to 6 cups (2½ to 3 pounds)
80	6 to 8 cups (3 to 4 pounds)

As with cats, an owner's final determination of how much to feed the dog should be based on the pet's overall reaction to feedings—weight rise or loss, pep, playfulness, vitality, etc.

To Streamline a Feline or Realign a Canine

Weight loss results, quite obviously, when the pet's food is restricted in some manner. Fasting is the best method to effect a desired and desirable weight loss, because it will result in cleansing the pet's system, detoxifying the animal and leaving it in a rejuvenated condition.

Diets low in starchy foods and high in leafy vegetables will also bring about a desired weight loss in pets, as will broth diets, fruit juice diets, fruit diets and raw milk, goat's milk or soy milk diets.

A seven-day streamlining and realigning menu might include:

1. Turnip greens, string beans and celery steamed together. Add 1 ounce raw beef and ½ cup grated raw celery.
2. Fresh corn, chard and broccoli steamed together. Add a raw egg yolk.
3. Spinach, peas, okra and peppers, steamed. An ounce of cottage cheese with chopped raw lettuce. Or nut butter (made by grinding raw nuts in a grinder or using the blender) in place of the cottage cheese.
4. Two bowls of raw milk, goat's milk or soy milk with ½ cup prune juice.
5. Two bowls of vegetable broth, with one raw egg yolk.
6. Steamed cabbage, peas and string beans. A very small amount of raw meat is optional.
7. Water, raw milk, soy milk *or* fruit juice with honey added.

Repeat the seven-day diet as long as it is felt to be necessary, and remember to give the pet exercise.

Pamper Your Pet's Palate with These Pleasing Pottages and Preparations

1. Make nut milk in the blender by mixing together 1 cup ground nuts, 2 cups pure water and 1 tablespoon honey. Use nut milk with cereals and other places where raw milk might be used.

2. Lay strips of cheddar cheese over steaming chopped string beans and carrots. Add ½ cup raw grated celery.

3. Prepare a pottage of whole potato, chopped celery, cabbage, string beans, and season it with an addition of small bits of raw beef.

4. Mix grated apples with ground nuts or nut butter.

5. Mix chopped cauliflower and squash with grated ricotta cheese.

6. Mix together 1 cup lima beans, 4 cups pure water, 1 cup sliced carrots, 1 cup pure vegetable oil (or nut butter), 1 pound okra, ½ onion, chopped, and ½ cup whole wheat flour. Steam for an hour or two, or until soft.

7. Mix mashed bananas and grated apples with 1 tablespoon honey and raw milk, cream or nut milk.

8. Place 1 pound whole wheat in 1 quart pure water and let stand overnight. Add 1 cup pure water and simmer for 3 hours. Serve with raw chopped vegetables, steamed vegetables or nut milk.

9. Add 3 cups pure water to 1 cup rice and simmer for 45 minutes. Add 2 cups grated celery, carrots and cabbage. Form into cakes and bake 15 minutes.

10. Add 1 cup raw milk to 2 cups whole oatmeal. Mix together and sprinkle with whole wheat flour. Cut into cakes and bake 15 minutes. Keep the cakes in a dry jar for several weeks.

Especially for Felines

1. Raw hamburger mixed with raw liver and okra.

2. Cheese melted over grated carrots.

3. Chopped raw fish mixed with steamed grated, chopped or sliced carrots.

4. Raw liver mixed with okra, peas and chopped string beans.
5. Steamed rice mixed with grated cheese.

Soul Food for Carnivorous Cats and Canines

1. Tripe fresh from the butcher, cleaned and mixed with fresh mashed yams, or chopped beet or carrot or celery tops.
2. Chitterlings fresh from the butcher, cleaned and mixed with fresh chopped turnip and/or collard greens.

Sample Pet Feeding Suggestions from Weaning to Four Months

8 A.M.	Raw milk or raw milk with prune juice or mashed prunes or raisins	Cereal flakes mixed with small amount of honey (1½ teaspoons to 3 tablespoons of flakes); soaked 10-15 minutes in raw milk
1 P.M.	Soaked oats or barley with vegetable broth or raw milk with raisins	½ cup raw meat mixed with 2 tablespoons raw chopped greens, parsley, celery tops, grated carrot
6 P.M.	Raw hamburger with 3 tablespoons grated carrot	Repeat 1 P.M. meal
11 P.M.	3 tablespoons raw meat, ½ teaspoon pure vegetable or nut oil, 1 teaspoon each grated celery, carrot and lettuce	½ cup raw milk and honey

On Sunday, do not feed until 1 P.M., and then begin with the cereal meal, giving only three feedings.

Sample Feedings from Four to Eight/Ten Months

	3 Feedings		2 Feedings
Morning	Raw milk with honey and ½ cup flaked barley or oats	1 P.M.	Cereal flakes, raw milk and honey
Noon	Raw milk with cottage cheese		
Night	Raw meat mixed with grated celery, lettuce or spinach; or steamed green vegetables	6-8 P.M.	Raw meat with mixed chopped raw vegetables

On Sunday, no food until the evening meal on both feeding schedules.

The chances are you won't be bringing any carnivorous, or "man-eating," plants into your home, so pure water, fresh air, sunlight and exercise are the main ingredients in a Natural Diet for Plants. Plants are living things, part of the order of creation, and have the needs and sensitivities of other living things. Jerry Baker, with whom I have appeared on the television talk-show circuit a few times, pinpointed this family relationship among living things in the title of his recent book, *Plants Are Like People.*

There are many interesting studies of the sensitivity of plants. I have been told, for example, that if a person kills a plant in a roomful of plants, all the other plants in the room will know and register a reaction whenever the killer walks into the room. Too bad plants can't talk! People who are worried about being mugged could carry a plant around with them to check out passersby!

All life needs the light from the sun, directly or indirectly, to survive. This is an important consideration in the positioning and arranging of house plants. When you see foliage on a plant bent over in one direction, it is a clear indication the plant is trying to get a peek at Mother Nature's sun. Small blooms, or no blooms at all, tall thin stems, and small pale leaves are further signs of an absence of sunlight.

Plants should be placed where they receive sunlight, and turned every few days so that all sides are exposed. A plant in a dark corner should be moved during certain periods of the day to get the benefit of the sunlight. If it can be placed outdoors, in a yard or patio, weather permitting, fine. If not, remember that the sunlight coming through a glass window is different from the direct light of the sun outdoors. The window should be open when the weather is favorable, or the sunlight filtered through a sheer curtain to prevent scorching of the leaves.

Pure fresh water is necessary for plants, rain water or melted snow being the best. Or spring water, but never tap water if it can be avoided. As Jerry Baker wisely reminds us, "Plants don't have teeth, so they can do without the fluoride!" So, of course, can the rest of us *with* teeth. During the winter months, three times or so, a natural vitamin (not chemical) capsule may be dissolved in a quart of pure water when watering plants. Plants need phosphate, carbon potassium or potash, and nitrogen for a balanced diet. They also need iron. Organic liquid substances rich in these ingredients may be fed to plants during growing season.

Along with giving plants outdoor exposure in the fresh air and sunlight on warm and mild days, Jerry Baker suggests exercise and shower baths. For exercise, place plants on top of the radio or stereo from time to time. The vibes keep the circulation moving and plants are music lovers anyway.

Finally, since the humidity in the average home is so low, plants wake up sharing the same feelings of the people who live there—

stopped-up noses, eyes stuck shut and dry mouths. A twice-a-month steam bath for plants is accomplished by placing a brick or block in the middle of a bucket and then placing the plant on top of it. Steaming water is added to the bottom of the bucket, taking care not to get any of the hot water on the plant or pot. Let the plant stand for five or six minutes. That, says Baker, constitutes a very welcome shower.

13

Cookin' with Mother Nature

I want to end this book as I began, by urging you to make *my* experience *your* experience of learning to live with Mother Nature.

It is so very, very important for the survival of America and Americans that *all* Americans look within themselves, recognize what they are doing to their bodies by improper eating habits, and then adopt a pattern of long life, health, happiness and brotherhood through proper nutrition.

The marks of insecurity are overweight and overeating. Folks who are insecure have a tendency to take out their insecurities on their own bodies. They raid the refrigerator, wipe out the pantry and empty the cookie jar, and think they are relieving their tensions by destroying their own bodies—those beautiful systems Mother Nature has provided.

I think one of the reasons we have so much overweight and overeating in these United States is that *America* is insecure. In her insecurity, America raids the refrigerator of Southeast Asia, wipes out the pantry of Latin America, munches and snacks on the freedom of peoples all over the world. And Americans themselves chew and gnaw at one another at home.

I believe diet is at the root of all problems. Americans who think so little of their own bodies that the average individual American consumes one hundred pounds of refined, "drugged" sugar each year will certainly allow the continued dropping of millions of tons of bombs on innocent people in Southeast Asia. Americans who consume billions of pounds of cigarettes will permit the continuation of a polluted system which spends billions of dollars on war and killing, and *makes* billions of dollars through the reckless pollution.

I have often said that the same *moral* pollution which keeps the Indian American locked up on the reservation keeps the smoke up in the air. If folks have so little respect for their own chests and lungs that they smoke cigarettes or make defective automobiles, filling the air with carbon monoxide fumes, how can they be expected to have respect for lakes, rivers and streams?

The same mentality which sanctions the dropping of bombs on Vietnam is responsible for spraying poisonous chemicals on the fruits and vegetables people eat. Even the rationale is the same. Spraying fruits and vegetables, it is said, is for the protection of the consumer. The same reasoning insists that bombing Vietnam is for the Vietnamese people's own good!

Just as individual Americans need to realize the beauty and marvel of their own bodies and clean out their systems, the national body must realize that its own system needs cleaning. America needs to go on a long purifying fast to realize it has one of the most beautiful systems the world has ever known—the United States Constitution—if Americans would only treat that system with respect and allow it to work as it was intended. And that realization and practice will only come when individual Americans start treating their *own* bodies with respect, cleaning both body and mind, and tuning in to the Universal Wisdom of Mother Nature.

As mentioned earlier, in the chapter on fasting, when the body is cleansed, the six basic fears plaguing humankind disappear. This is true of both individuals and nations. America seems to be afraid the nation will be overwhelmed *externally*, by some mysterious force—a red menace, a yellow peril, etc. It never seems to occur to America that the greatest menace is *internal*, the gradual and not so mysterious degeneration of the bodies of Americans and the effect that disintegration has on the mind, emotions and behavior patterns.

Individual Americans show the same irrational fears. Some worry and fret while riding in an airplane, fearing the possibility that the plane will crash. It never occurs to them there is more danger in the meal they eat on the plane. When the basic fears disappear as a result of cleansing the system, the terrible problems rooted in those basic fears also begin to be solved—racial hatreds, bigotry and misunderstanding, an infatuation with war and killing—all of the seemingly "insoluble" problems we face today.

I long to see the day when a "fearless" America will be so cleansed and enlightened and so in tune with Mother Nature that *real* solutions to human problems will be offered. Two of the great problems facing America today are alcoholism and drug addiction. And I am sure a change in diet and a cleansing of the body are the way to treat both addictions.

Drugs, so-called stimulants, are really depressants; these include tobacco, hard narcotics, coffee, commercial tea and all kinds of pills. There is a *feeling* of stimulation because the body rouses itself to get rid of the poison. That's the quick energy stimulants give. It is the same way the body deals with meat-eating. No stimulant "imparts strength" any more than digging a spur into the side of a horse "imparts strength" to the poor animal. It may cause it to run faster, or cause energy to be *expended* more rapidly.

So a change in diet and a cleansing of the system would quite naturally be a logical and long-term way to treat addiction. The more the body gets back to its normal condition, the less the desire for false and destructive stimulations.

In the Sermon on the Mount, Jesus, one of Mother Nature's greatest spokesmen, said: "You are the salt of the earth. But if the salt has lost its taste, how shall its saltness be restored?" Today's chemists and so-called experts would answer, "Throw in some potassium iodide and put it back on the shelf." But Jesus was talking about restoration, restored human beings, new folks whose "taste" was restored in fullness. People of good taste, in other words.

Rather than complete restoration, we see today an increased reliance upon another drug or chemical solution to the problem of narcotics addiction. The replacement of heroin with methadone seems to be gaining increased acceptance. Not everyone agrees with this kind of transferral of dependencies, and a New York City commissioner resigned not too long ago in protest against the increasing obsession with methadone as a solution. The point is that such solutions represent the "put it back on the shelf" type of thinking. Give them another drug rather than a restored and renewed body.

As a veteran occupant of some of the nation's most prestigious jails, I think the jails and prisons of America would be a perfect place to initiate dietary reform and nutritional rehabilitation. In the jails are many addicts and others suffering from mental disturbances and emotional hostilities which could be corrected by dietary reform. If prisons are what they claim to be, centers of rehabilitation, then the released prisoner could leave with a new body and a new mind—a really new lease on life.

Penal systems in every state should bring in honest, ethical nutritional experts to guide and counsel a change in jailhouse menus. In jail, a person is under ideal conditions for trying dietary reform, not being tempted by the bad food available out in the streets.

Jail menus should have fresh fruit juices at every breakfast, fresh fruit or raw salad for lunch, and dinners composed 80 percent of raw salad. Meat should be cut down to a bare minimum, served only on weekends if at all, for all those who wish to take part in this worthy enterprise.

Such dietary reform would cut down not only on food expenditures in the jails but also on medical expenses. Classes should be given to teach prisoners the workings of the body and the importance of proper nutrition and elimination. As they begin to look and feel better, much of the resentment now directed toward the typical jailhouse menu would fade away.

In any event the commissaries in jails should offer more health food—sunflower seeds, pumpkin seeds, almonds, filberts, oranges, fresh fruits and the like—in place of, or in addition to, candy and pastries. Prisoners should be encouraged to purchase lemons and honey and make lemonade, instead of loading up on sodas and other artificial drinks. The jail should provide blenders for this purpose. Every jailhouse kitchen should be supplied with adequate juicing equipment. Enema bags should be available for every prisoner in every cell who wants one.

Fasting should also be encouraged. I personally feel it should be rewarded. Prisoners who engage in purifying fasts could be credited with good-behavior time. Prisoners should be encouraged to experiment with a day of fruit, a day of fruit juice and a day of water. And at the end of such a period of body attention, the prisoner should be given a day of rest from work.

The penal system which initiates these suggestions just might

find it is on top of a tremendous breakthrough in the area of rehabilitation. It just might find that difficulties in rehabilitation stem
more from the jailhouse kitchen than from any other source.

A truly "fearless" America, cleansed and renewed, would take
the lead not only in *feeding* the world but in providing *nutrition* for the world. United States foreign aid would encourage
small nations to work cooperatively in doing research into the
truly nutritious foods and to become manufacturers and suppli-
ers of the world's health needs—much as tiny Japan has become
the supplier of the world's desire for gadgets. There are so many
foods, principally sea products, that are at the very top of the
nutritional ladder—kelp, Irish moss, dulse, agar, sesame seeds,
sunflower seeds, soybeans, brewer's yeast, wheat germ, almonds,
pumpkin seeds, celery, carrots, dates, honey, oranges, lemons,
limes, cabbage (green and red), tomatoes, squash seeds and all
dried fruits. Yet much emphasis is placed on supplying meat and
milk and other animal products to so-called underprivileged nations; teaching cattle-raising techniques and providing expertise
in dairy farming. Foreign aid should take a cue from India and
let the cows alone.

Let me close with this final word. The more you live in Mother
Nature's kitchen, the more you will be blessed with the true re-
wards in life. Mother Nature provides what we are supposed to
have. And we get a clue from the reaction of her creatures to what
is right for us and what is wrong.

Anything we are supposed to have Mother Nature places at
our doorstep. At twelve noon, we walk out the door and we know
where Mother Nature's sun will be. Her rain comes down to us,
and her air and her wind. But birds fly away when we approach
and animals scamper at the sound of our footsteps. It's as though
they know we can't be trusted.

Apples don't run away from us. They fall off the trees into our waiting hands. Oranges, pears and peaches don't try to escape. They remain in Mother Nature's kitchen, being baked and ripened by her natural sunlight. So enjoy her pantry! You'll be so glad you did. Because Mother Nature's cookin', baby!

Peace be with you.

Acknowledgments

I want to thank Jeannette Hopkins for her editorial wisdom and humanitarian patience in seeing this book through to its completion. She always finds a way to make it possible to meet deadlines and make production schedules!

Thanks over and over again to Jim Sanders and his brilliant comedy mind. You will find his wit and humor scattered throughout these pages. I also want to thank Jim's wife, Jackie, and his daughter, Jennifer, for their contribution in keeping him in happy spirits.

A word of deep appreciation to Jim McGraw, Francis Johnson and Elaine Shepherd for their help in the preparation of the manuscript. I'd also like to acknowledge the special support of all my endeavors given to me by Adam D. Bourgeois, James Black, Mike Watley, Bernie Kleinman, Dick Shelton, Steve Jaffe, Kevin Eggers, Paul Shelton, Warren St. James, Garland Gregory, George O'Hare of Sears, Roebuck, Bob Walker of American Program Bureau in Boston, Bob Johnson of *Jet* magazine and Ralph Mann, Marvin Josephson, Bob Chuck and Marge Casciello of International Famous Agency in New York City.

Part of the period of preparing this manuscript was spent on the beautiful island of Jamaica. I'd like to publicly express my gratitude and personal admiration to Prime Minister Michael

Manley, and his lovely wife, Beverly, and to Senator Dudley J. Thompson, minister of state.

I hope all these good friends (and relatives) listed above will soon join me in a life of cookin' with Mother Nature.

This book bears the strong imprint of two very natural folks who keep me in close touch with Mother Nature—Dr. Alvenia M. Fulton, whose wisdom, insight and menus are contained in these pages, and naprapath Dr. Roland J. Sidney of Chicago, my family's doctor.

Finally, a word of love and gratitude to my own natural household: my wife, Lillian, and the kids—Michele, Lynne, Pamela, Paula, Stephanie, Gregory, Miss, Christian and Ayanna.

Bibliography

Raw Food Diet

Benjamin, Harry. *Commonsense Vegetarianism*. London: Lewes Press, Wightman & Co. Ltd., 1950.

Bernard, R. W. *Organic Foods for Health*. Mokelumne Hill, California: Health Research, 1956.

Carrington, Hereward. *The Hygienic Way of Life: The Argument for Vegetarianism*. Mokelumne Hill, California: Health Research, 1957.

Haffenden, Alfred Hy. *Systems of Feeding*. Essex, England: The C. W. Daniel Company, 1953.

Thomas, Julian P. *The Advantages of Raw Food*. Mokelumne Hill, California: Health Research, 1956.

Tobe, John H. *"No Cook" Book*. St. Catharines, Ontario: The Provoker Press, 1969.

Walker, N. W. *Diet and Salad Suggestions*. Phoenix, Arizona: Norwalk Press, 1940.

The Use of Fresh Raw Juices

Clinkard, C. E. *The Uses of Juices*. London: Whitcombe and Tombs Ltd., 1960.

Kirschner, H. E. *Live Food Juices*. Monrovia, California: H. E. Kirschner Publications, 1957.

Lust, John B. *About Raw Juices*. London: Thorsons Publishers Ltd., 1962.

Newman, Laura. *Make Your Juicer Your Drug Store*. New York: Benedict Lust Publications, 1970.

Walker, N. W. *Raw Vegetable Juices: What's Missing in Your Body*. Phoenix, Arizona: Norwalk Press, 1936.

Disease and Natural Healing

Airola, Paavo O. *There Is a Cure for Arthritis*. West Nyack, New York: Parker Publishing Company, Inc., 1968.

Bragg, Paul C. *Toxicless Diet Body Purification and Healing System*. Burbank, California: Health Science, 1967.

Harris, Ben Charles. *Kitchen Medicines*. New York: Pocket Books, 1970.

Kloss, Jethro. *Back to Eden*. New York: Benefician Books, 1971.

Page, Melvin E. *Body Chemistry in Health and Disease*. St. Petersburg, Florida: The Page Foundation, 1968.

Ramacharaka, Yogi. *The Practical Water Cure*. Chicago: The Yogi Publication Society, 1937.

Taylor, Lillian. *Clean Up the Blood Stream and Live.* Mokelumne Hill, California: Health Research, 1944.

Tilden, J. H. *Toxemia Explained.* Denver: The World Press, Inc., 1926.

Walker, N. W. *Become Younger.* Phoenix, Arizona: Norwalk Press, 1949.

Warmbrand, Max. *The Encyclopedia of Natural Health.* Brooklyn, N.Y.: Groton Press, 1962.

Fasting

Bragg, Paul C. *The Miracle of Fasting.* Burbank, California: Health Science, 1969.

Buchinger, Otto H. F. *The Fasting Story, Number One.* Mokelumne Hill, California: Health Research, 1962.

————. *Everything You Want to Know About Fasting.* New York: Pyramid Books, 1972.

Carrington, Hereward. *Save Your Life by Fasting.* St. Catharines, Ontario: The Provoker Press, 1969.

Hanoka, N. S. *Scientific Fasting and Natural Living.* Diyatalawa, Ceylon: Natural Health Publications, 1953.

Hazzard, Linda B. *About Scientific Fasting.* New York: Benedict Lust Publications, 1967.

Jaffrey, Kenneth S. *How to Fast.* Townsville, Australia: T. Willmett & Sons, Ltd., 1967.

Purinton, Edward Earle. *The Philosophy of Fasting.* 1906. Reprint. Mokelumne Hill, California: Health Research, n.d.

Smith, Frederick W. *Journal of a Fast.* New York: Ballantine Books, 1972.

Wade, Carlson. *The Natural Way to Health Through Controlled Fasting.* New York: Arc Books, Inc., 1968.

Child and Baby Care

Davis, Adelle. *Let's Have Healthy Children.* New York: Harcourt, Brace, Jovanovich, Inc., 1959.

Rotondi, Pietro. *Your Vegetarian Baby.* Hollywood, California: n.p., 1954.

Pet and Plant Care

Baker, Jerry. *Plants Are Like People.* New York: Pocket Books, 1972.

Kireluk, Bernice. *Let's Raise Healthy Dogs Naturally.* St. Catharines, Ontario: The Provoker Press, 1970.

Miller, Harry. *The Common Sense Book of Puppy and Dog Care.* New York: Bantam Books, 1956.

———. *The Common Sense Book of Kitten and Cat Care.* New York: Bantam Books, 1966.

Ogden, Donald I. *Natural Care of Pets.* Mokelumne Hill, California: Health Research, 1959.

Further Sources

Burton, Maurice. *University Dictionary of Mammals of the World*. New York: Thomas Y. Crowell Company, 1962.

Carque, Otto. *The Key to Rational Dietetics*. Mokelumne Hill, California: Health Research, 1966.

Conason, Emil G., and Metz, Ella. *The Salt-Free Diet Cookbook*. New York: Grosset & Dunlap, 1949.

Godlovitch, Stanley and Rosalind, and Harris, John, eds. *Animals, Men and Morals*. New York: Taplinger Publishing Company, 1972.

Gregory, Dick. *The Shadow That Scares Me*. New York: Doubleday & Co., 1968.

———. *Dick Gregory's Political Primer*. New York: Harper & Row, 1972.

Hauser, Gayelord. *The Gayelord Hauser Cook Book*. New York: Capricorn Books, 1963.

Heritage, Ford. *Composition and Facts About Foods*. Mokelumne Hill, California: Health Research, 1968.

Hoffman, Bob. *How Good Is the American Diet?* York, Pennsylvania: York Barbell Company, 1965.

Macia, Rafael. *The Natural Foods and Nutrition Handbook*. New York: Perennial Library, Harper & Row, 1972.

Morishita, K. *Milk*. Los Angeles: The Ohsawa Foundation, n.d.

Muir, Ada. *Food in Relation to Health*. St. Paul, Minnesota: Llewellyn Publications, 1966.

Rodale, J. I. *The Encyclopedia for Healthful Living.* Emmaus, Pennsylvania: Rodale Books, Inc., 1960.

———. *The Complete Book of Food and Nutrition.* Emmaus, Pennsylvania: Rodale Books, Inc., 1972.

Tobe, John H. *Eat Right and Be Healthy.* St. Catharines, Ontario: Modern Publications Reg'd, 1964.

Wade, Carlson. *Magic Minerals: Key to Better Health.* West Nyack, New York: Parker Publishing Company, Inc., 1967.

Index

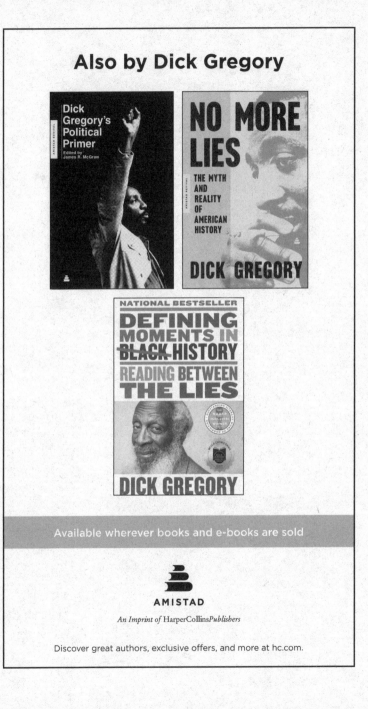